SEN 2 REVISION BOOK

CASE STUDIES AND OBJECTIVE TEST QUESTIONS

Edited and compiled by
LYNN COPCUTT SRN DN (London) RNT. B.Ed. (Hons).
Senior Tutor, Queen Elizabeth School of Nursing,
Edgbaston, Birmingham.

PASTEST SERVICE
Hemel Hempstead
Hertfordshire England

© 1983 PASTEST SERVICE
P.O. Box 81, Hemel Hempstead, Hertfordshire.
Tel: 0442 - 52113

First published 1983

ISBN 0-906896-11-8

British Library Cataloguing in Publication Data

Copcutt, Lynn
SEN 2: case histories and objective test questions
for pupil nurses.
1. Nursing - Problems, exercises, etc
I. Title
610.73'076   RT55

ISBN 0-906896-11-8

Text prepared using Sirius 1 microcomputer.
Phototypeset by Designed Publications using an interface.
Printed by Martins of Berwick.

CONTENTS

Brackets indicate the number of case studies in each subject. Each case study has 4 related questions.

NOTES TO THE READER

This book has been produced to assist pupil nurses preparing for the multiple choice paper for the General Roll, established by the General Nursing Council for England and Wales.

All examinations create anxiety for candidates. Multiple choice questions can pose particular difficulties for some people either because of lack of experience in attempting this type of test, or because previously they have been faced with questions which bear little similarity to those found in the actual examination. I therefore feel there is a need for this book and its sister edition for student nurses, because they contain carefully selected, pre-tested and validated questions specifically intended to prepare the learner nurse for the amended GNC State Final Assessment which begins in January 1983.

Practising nurse teachers were invited to submit questions for consideration. Over 300 case studies containing 1,200 questions were scrutinized to obtain the 240 questions finally accepted. After initial editing the questions were compiled into test papers of approximately 100 questions each. These tests were taken by a minimum of 100 finalist pupil nurses in more than 60 schools of nursing throughout the country.

Computer analysis followed and only those questions meeting predetermined levels of difficulty and discrimination were considered for inclusion. In addition, comments received from pupil nurses and teaching staff participating with the pre-testing of questions were considered. Thank you all for your co-operation.

The preparation of multiple choice tests is not easy, but every attempt has been made to ensure that this publication will become a helpful part of the arduous task of examination revision.

This book contains 240 multiple choice questions, 180 of which are compiled into 45 case studies each with 4 questions. The remaining 60 questions are grouped together as a practice examination consisting of 7 case studies and 32 individual questions, grouped together in order to cover the range of topics and degree of difficulty the pupil nurse is likely to meet.

Each question consists of an initial statement followed by four alternative answers, marked A B C D. Only *one* of these is correct.

Notes to the reader

Questions are printed on the right-hand page, with the correct answers and explanations on the following page. Alongside each answer you will find a percentage figure which indicates the number of finalist nurses who chose the correct answer during pre-testing of the questions. Questions with a high percentage are easier than those with a low percentage. By using this information you will be able to identify areas which need concentrated revision. It will also enable you to assess your own level of performance compared to that of other finalists. Attempt each question before you look at the answers, this is the best way to test your knowledge and to highlight strengths and weaknesses.

Finally, a word of thanks to the many people who have assisted with the preparation of this book especially my husband Ian who has been of immeasurable support and provided encouragement in times of need.

L.C.

NOTES FOR GENERAL GUIDANCE

1. In the General Nursing Council Examination the multiple choice questions are printed in booklet form with about 8 questions to the page. Be prepared for the fact that the print is fairly small, sometimes this comes as rather a surprise to candidates and is enough initially to jar their concentration.

2. Choose whichever of the four distractors you feel is correct and do not worry or be put off if you seem to have, for example, four "B" correct answers in a row. This is perfectly possible, have the courage of your convictions.

3. Remember that you can change your mind and alter your answer on the computer sheet. However, having done this it is *impossible* to return to your original choice of answer. So think carefully before committing yourself. Once done, leave that question and move on to the next.

4. When revising do not just sit passively reading books and lecture notes, but remember that many multiple choice questions will test your ability to reason. Therefore, when revising, try to understand *why* nursing care and observations are carried out, and their significance.
   Questions which test your ability to reason or your understanding of nursing care could ask:

   > Which one of the following is the *reason* why a patient with chronic bronchitis is prescribed a low-concentration of oxygen?

   or

   > A patient with dyspnoea is nursed in the upright position *because.......*

   A question testing your memory only could be as follows:

   > Which of the following patients rely on a lowered oxygen level in order to stimulate respiration? The patient suffering from
   >
   > A   pneumonia
   > B   chronic bronchitis
   > C   pneumothorax
   > D   bronchiectasis

   When revising, instead of saying to yourself "the patient following cholecystectomy will need chest physiotherapy" you ought really to be asking yourself "why does the patient following cholecystectomy need chest physiotherapy?". Similarly, instead of "the patient with hypertension may need renal investigations" try "why does the hypertensive patient need renal investigations?". This will give an added depth to your revision and will most certainly enhance your chances of success in the multiple choice examination.

Here are some more examples of revision questions:

Why does the patient with pneumonia complain of pain on inspiration?

Why does constipation predispose to the development of diverticular disease?

Why is a high protein diet prescribed for a patient with nephrotic syndrome?

Why is a t-tube clamped prior to removal?

Why, if the victim is shocked, should a light cover only be used at the scene of an accident?

Why does albuminuria contribute to the formation of oedema?

Why do patients need bed- rest following a myocardial infarction?

Why is oxygen humidified?

5. If all else fails and you simply cannot work out the correct answer to any particular question *always* attempt the question and choose one of the four alternatives. Marks are not deducted for wrong answers therefore you have nothing to lose.

   In the Final Examination *always attempt every question.*

6. Work methodically through the test reading only *one* question at a time. Try to work out the answer but if you cannot, *leave a space* on the computer answer sheet and move on to the next question.

7. Check carefully throughout the test that you are marking your answer in the correct space on the computer answer sheet.

8. Having worked through the test once, return to questions you left earlier and attempt to answer them. If all else fails, guess!

9. On completion of the test, check that your candidate number is entered correctly and leave. It is not generally advisable to go back to the beginning of the test checking every answer as this could cause you to make rushed last minute alterations which cannot then be re-corrected.

10. If you can, avoid the temptation to discuss your answers with your colleagues afterwards since this will add to your anxiety. Questions are seldom remembered accurately, so it is far better to wait patiently for results day!

Good Luck.

REVISION CHECKLIST

Notes for using the Revision Checklist.

You will see, in the left-hand coloumn, a list of topics for revision, under 4 headings:-

> Patients who are ....
> Patients who have ....
> First Aid.
> Special needs of children.
> Special needs of the elderly.

Take each topic in turn, and read ALONG the page where you will find 4 empty columns. This means that each topic in the left-hand column ought to be revised in 4 stages and ticks placed in the appropriate columns on completion.

	Actual problems	Potential problems	Nursing care plan & observations	Treatment/ investigations Drugs/ Therapeutic
Patients who are breathless	✓	✓	✓	✓
Patients who are pyrexial	✓	✓	✓	✓

e.g. Whilst revising care of the patient who is pyrexial, you should have covered a wide range of previous material:-

1. Anxiety faced by patient and family, and how best to help.

2. Risk of dehydration.

3. Methods of lowering body temparature, and their hazards. Keeping pyrexial patients cool, dry and comfortable. The need for mouth and skin care.
    Accurate observation of temperature, pulse, respiration rate. Special signs needing immediate treatment/reporting.

4. Common causes of pyrexia and their treatment.
    Drugs used to lower temperature and their hazards.

REVISION TOPICS	Actual problems	Potential problems	Nursing care plan & observations	Treatment/ investigations Drugs/ Therapeutic
Patients who are				
Newly admitted				
Breathless				
Oedematous				
Incontinent of urine				
Incontinent of faeces				
Paralysed				
Bedfast				
Infested				
Unconscious				
Emaciated				
Obese				
Pyrexial				
Vomiting				
Awaiting surgery				
Returning from surgery				
In plaster or traction				
Unable to eat				
Constipated				
Bleeding - externally				
- internally				
Shocked				
Blind				
Deaf				
Jaundiced				
Dying				
Patients who have				
Wounds and drains				
Stomas				
Nasogastric tubes				
Indwelling catheters				
Chest drains				
Fits				
Infusions/transfusions				
Accidents				
Pain				
Restricted mobility				
Insomnia				
Infections				
Respiratory disorders				
Cardiovascular disorders				

Revision checklist

	Actual problems	Potential problems	Nursing care plan & observations	Treatment/ investigations Drugs/ Therapeutic
(cont.)				

Alimentary disorders
Endocrine disorders
Locomotor disorders
Renal disorders
Neurological disorders
ENT disorders
Reproductive system
    disorders
Skin disorders
Malignant disorders

First Aid:

Resuscitation
Heamorrhage
Shock
Asphyxia
Fractures
Burns/scalds
Poisoning
Fits
Ward accidents &
Emergencies

**Special needs of
children:**

e.g. play
     security
     diet
     sleep/rest
     parents

**Special needs of
the elderly:**

e.g. dignity
     independence
     individuality
     continence
     diet
     mobility
     communication
     rehabilitation

RESPIRATION

On each of the following pages you will find a case study followed by 4 related questions. Answers are overleaf.

Mr Brown is a 75 year old man who lives in a small terraced house. He has suffered with recurring chest problems for many years and he is now admitted to a medical ward with an acute exacerbation of chronic bronchitis.

1. Which of the following describes an acute exacerbation of chronic bronchitis? A

   A further narrowing of the bronchial tree
   B superimposed infection on already damaged respiratory passages
   C sudden dramatic increased tidal volume
   D substantial decrease in sputum production

2. Which of the following is the *best* description of dyspnoea:

   A being aware of greater effort needed for respiration
   B a sensation of sharp pain on taking a deep breath
   C greater difficulty in breathing when lying flat
   D difficulty in breathing when eating solid foods

3. Which of the following is the cause of cyanosis:

   A increase in the proportion of white to red blood cells
   B increase in the alkalinity of the blood
   C low carbon dioxide levels in the plasma
   D deficiency in the oxygenation of erythrocytes

4. Which of the following should be used to counteract Mr Brown's severe cyanosis:

   A polymask continuously
   B oxygen tent intermittently
   C nasal cannulae intermittently
   D ventimask continuously

Answers overleaf

Answers and explanations

1. B 65%

Chronic bronchitis is a chronic disease of the respiratory passages. An acute chest infection in addition to the longstanding lung damage is known as an acute exacerbation of chronic bronchitis. (To exacerbate means to make worse.)

2. A 61%

Strictly speaking, dyspnoea means difficulty experienced with breathing so options A, B, C and D could be correct. However the question asked for the *best* description, which is A.

3. D 72%

Cyanosis is a blueness of the lips, fingernails and skin and is always caused by a lack of oxygen in the red blood cells, not A, B or C.

4. D 31%

Mr Brown has carbon dioxide levels in his bloodstream which are above normal limits because his chronic lung disease impairs diffusion of gases in the alveoli. For the same reason his oxygen levels are low, resulting in cyanosis. When administering oxygen it is important to use a ventimask delivering air and oxygen. Thus, whilst cyanosis is relieved, the blood levels do not alter too dramatically which might cause the respiratory centre in the brain not to respond, thereby impairing breathing even more.

A young football fan, 17 years old, is accidentally stabbed. The knife is lodged in the right anterior chest wall as he collapses on the ground in pain, but conscious.

5. Which of the following actions is the correct first aid procedure:

    A   remove the knife and apply a pressure pad
    B   lie the patient flat to prevent shock
    C   apply a supportive dressing around the knife
    D   apply a constrictive bandage to keep the chest wall still

6. Which of the following positions will facilitate the casualty's breathing:

    A   supine
    B   semi-recumbent
    C   recovery
    D   left lateral

7. Which of the following will a pneumothorax and haemothorax cause:

    A   slow pulse and respiration
    B   dyspnoea and cyanosis
    C   raised pulse and blood pressure
    D   immediate cardiac arrest

8. What is the purpose of an underwater seal drain? To

    A   allow the lung to rest and recover
    B   allow air to enter the lung for respiration
    C   prevent air escaping from the lung
    D   allow re-expansion of the collapsed lung

Answers overleaf

5. **C 59%**

Removal of the knife may cause further damage thereby increasing the risk to the casualty's life. The knife should be supported by a clean, preferably sterile dressing in order to prevent further injury, to stop air entry to the pleura, and to reduce the risk of infection.

6. **B 54%**

With a painful injured chest wall the casualty has difficulty in breathing. The semi-recumbent position is more helpful as good expansion of the chest is made easier.

7. **B 59%**

Haemothorax and pneumothorax result in collapse of one lung. The casualty will develop dyspnoea and become cyanosed as gas exchange is reduced because only one lung will be functioning normally.

8. **D 79%**

A water seal drain allows the lung to re-expand as air and blood drain away from the pleural space. The water seal prevents air and fluid being drawn into the pleural space from the drainage bottle as long as the tubing remains intact and the drainage bottle is kept below the level of the bed.

John Longden, aged 72 years, has hypostatic pneumonia and is unable to get out of bed without help due to multiple sclerosis.

9. Which of the following is the *main* reason for frequently turning Mr Longden? To

    A   prevent contraction deformity
    B   facilitate expectoration and coughing
    C   increase his muscular strength
    D   prevent urinary retention and infection

10. Which of the following *best* explains why Mr Longden developed pneumonia:

    A   secretions form an ideal culture medium
    B   his resistance to infection is no longer effective
    C   there is reduced white cell production
    D   resistance to antibiotics occurs easily

11. Which of the following is the *most* likely way of ensuring drainage of the respiratory passages:

    A   pleural aspiration
    B   bronchoscopy and suction
    C   bronchial lavage
    D   postural drainage

12. How should Mr Longden's pyrexia be reduced? By

    A   keeping the room temperature static
    B   sponging of the skin
    C   application of ice packs
    D   administration of chlorpromazine

Answers overleaf

9. **B** 76%

If the patient is allowed to remain in one position for long periods he is likely to develop pressure sores, and a chest infection due to secretions collecting in the lungs and becoming infected. Regular turning ensures good drainage from the lungs and makes it easier for Mr Longden to expectorate the infected sputum.

10. **A** 17%

The collected secretions form a culture medium which is moist, warm and nutritious in which bacteria thrive and multiply rapidly.

11. **D** 84%

Where a cough is productive it is important to encourage expectoration. Each lung lobe should be emptied with the patient in the best possible position as when postural drainage is carried out. This is therefore the *most* likely method. Option A would remove fluid from the pleural space only, not the respiratory passages. Options B and C are unlikely.

12. **B** 55%

Frequent sponging of the skin will reduce Mr Longden's pyrexia but care must be taken to ensure that a gradual reduction occurs, not a very sudden change which could shock the patient.

Mr Martin, aged 78 years, has been admitted with an acute exacerbation of his chronic bronchitis. He is in an anxious state worrying about his invalid wife at home.

13. Which of the following will *best* aid expectoration of secretions:

    A   regular linctus as prescribed
    B   nurse in an upright position
    C   oxygen given via a ventimask
    D   an adequate fluid intake

14. Which of the following observations are *most* significant:

    A   sputum colour and 4 hourly temperature
    B   fluid intake and output
    C   anxiety level and pulse rate
    D   state of mouth and fluid intake

15. Which of the following should be a priority once the acute phase is over:

    A   sit him up and loosen his clothing
    B   make arrangements for his wife's care
    C   give him inhalations as necessary
    D   take a full history of his family

16. Which of the following complications may Mr Martin develop:

    A   left sided heart failure
    B   right sided heart failure
    C   mitral valve incompetence
    D   subacute bacterial endocarditis

Answers overleaf

13. **D   61%**

By preventing dehydration expectoration will be easier for Mr Martin because the secretions in his respiratory passages will be moist. If he became dehydrated the water from the sputum would be reabsorbed making it viscous and hard to expectorate. Linctus depresses the cough reflex and using the upright position or oxygen therapy does not directly aid sputum expectoration.

14. **A   53%**

All the observations are significant, however because of the acute chest infection which is superimposed on top of his chronic bronchitis, sputum colour and temperature recordings are *most* significant in order to detect response to antibiotic therapy and improvement in the acute condition.

15. **B   43%**

Option A should already have been done to aid breathing in the acute phase. Options C and D may be carried out but are not always necessary. Option B is correct as Mr Martin is worried about his wife and as she is an invalid it is important to make arrangements for her care.

16. **B   41%**

Chronic bronchitis results in some degree of permanent lung damage (emphysema). Alteration in the function of the lungs can result in excessive strain on the right ventricle which is responsible for pumping blood via the pulmonary arteries to the lungs. Right sided heart failure will result in congestive cardiac failure. Heart disease secondary to disease of the lungs is known as cor pulmonale.

Michael, a 17 year old adolescent, is admitted as an emergency accompanied by his worried parents. After examination the doctor diagnoses a severe attack of acute asthma.

17. Which of the following will relieve the bronchospasm:

    A suxamethonium
    B diazepam
    C adrenaline
    D Intal (sodium cromoglycate)

18. Why may steroids be given? Because primarily they

    A reduce the risk of infection
    B increase available energy
    C enhance the allergic response
    D relieve inflamed bronchial membrane

19. Which of the following will be advised prior to discharge:

    A stay indoors to avoid allergens
    B move to a warmer climate
    C take a prescribed prophylactic drug regularly
    D take a rest and holiday in the country

20. Michael will *best* be re-assured during the acute attack by

    A the nurse who quickly tries to relieve his symptoms
    B a calm, efficient and confident manner
    C an explanation of the procedures to be performed
    D listening to him talk about his feelings of fear

Answers overleaf

17. **C   9%**

Where spasm of the bronchial muscle narrows the lumen (size of opening) of the airways a bronchodilator drug such as adrenaline is prescribed to relax them. Thus the lumen dilates and makes breathing easier. Option D is given to prevent bronchospasm by inhibiting the allergic reaction, it is not a bronchodilator.

18. **D   84%**

Steroids have an anti-allergic and anti-inflammatory action, hence their value in cases of acute asthma. They are life-saving drugs but prescribed with caution because of the large number of side effects which may arise and the necessity to wean a patient off them gradually.

19. **C   84%**

To avoid further distressing attacks Michael will be prescribed a prophylactic drug such as sodium cromoglycate (Intal) which should be taken frequently as prescribed to prevent an attack. Young people may be reluctant to take medication if they feel well, so its importance should be emphasised. (Prophylaxis means prevention of disease or preventive treatment.)

20. **B   56%**

Michael is afraid because he is unable to breathe and feels as if he is suffocating. The nurse who is calm and knows what she needs to do will help to reduce his fear. He will have no energy to talk or listen to explanations of future procedures.

Mrs Lane, a 59 year old widow with bronchial carcinoma, has had a lobectomy. Mrs Lane is very depressed about her recent bereavement and medical diagnosis.

21. Which of the following should be done by the nurse:

    A   explain the tumour and the prognosis of surgery
    B   tell the patient she will be better soon
    C   listen to Mrs Lane's fears and memories
    D   tell her not to worry and try to be more positive

22. Which of the following is the *most* important care of the underwater seal drain? To

    A   measure the amount of drainage daily
    B   encourage deep breathing hourly
    C   prevent air entering the thoracic cavity
    D   observe the "swinging" in the drainage tube

23. When is the water seal drain removed:

    A   on the 3rd post-operative day
    B   when no air bubbles escape from the tube
    C   if fluid drainage begins to increase
    D   after X-ray indicates the lung has re-expanded

24. Which of the following methods of drain removal is correct:

    A   exert a sharp pull to remove it quickly
    B   remove the tube and seal the opening
    C   remove the tube and apply a light dressing
    D   shorten the tube daily before removal

Answers overleaf

Answers and explanations

21. **C 83%**

In order to give Mrs Lane the best chance to come to terms with her
bereavement and diagnosis the nurse should give her the opportunity
to talk to a person who is prepared to listen.

22. **C 80%**

The water seal is applied to the chest drain to prevent air from
entering the thoracic cavity. If it becomes dislodged the wound
should immediately have a sealing dressing applied. If the tube
becomes detached from the water seal it should be clamped thus
preventing air entry and further collapse of the remaining lung.

23. **D 80%**

The water seal drain is to allow drainage of air and fluid, prevent
compression of the lung and allow re-expansion. An X-ray is taken if
drainage is reduced to nil and if expansion has occurred the drain is
removed.

24. **B 24%**

The nurse removes the tube by using a pad prepared with sterile
vaseline gauze, or something similar, to form an airtight seal. An
alternative method is for the doctor to apply a suture which is drawn
tight on removal of the tube. Prior to removal of the tube the patient is
asked to breathe in and hold her breath, the tube is then quickly
removed.

Mr Jones is 72 years old and is admitted cyanosed and dyspnoeic. He is very distressed as is his wife who accompanies him. He has a long - standing history of chronic bronchitis.

25. Which of the following approaches with the oxygen mask would be *best*:

   A   establish a good relationship and introduce the mask
   B   put the mask on quietly to avoid distress
   C   explain clearly to the patient and apply the mask
   D   apply the mask before turning on the oxygen

26. How is the benefit obtained from bronchodilators assessed? By

   A   quantity and colour of sputum
   B   level of exercise tolerance
   C   recording the rate and depth of respiration
   D   recording the before and after Peak Expiratory Flow

27. Which of the following should the patient be advised on discharge:

   A   keep windows open to ensure good ventilation
   B   sleep in a warm atmosphere
   C   take regular exercise to keep fit
   D   continue trips to the cinema or football matches

28. Which of the following will *most* effectively reduce Mrs Jones anxiety:

   A   show a caring attitude and give simple explanations
   B   advise Mrs Jones to return at visiting time when her husband will be feeling better
   C   suggest the doctor gives her a tranquillizer
   D   arrange for a cup of tea and tell her all will be well

25. **A   27%**

Many patients are afraid of the oxygen mask as they feel it "enclosing them" producing a sense of suffocation which may cause a feeling of panic. If the patient trusts the nurse and has a good relationship with her, he will accept the mask more easily which is essential to relieve his oxygen lack. Whilst B, C and D are all possible, option A is the best.

26. **D   79%**

When a bronchodilator drug is given in obstructive airway disease the patient's Peak Expiratory Flow should be recorded before and after treatment. If benefit does not occur a need for a change in treatment may be indicated.

27. **B   29%**

On discharge the patient should be advised to avoid crowded places where infection may be picked up, take exercise within the limits of his respiratory capacity and sleep in a warm atmosphere as cold air may cause constriction of the bronchi.

28. **A   81%**

The nurse's attitude of caring and giving simple explanations will reduce anxiety caused by fear and lack of knowledge. Whilst option D may help, it will not be as effective as A.

Simon, aged 16, is brought into casualty with an acute asthmatic attack. He is on his own as his parents have gone out for the evening.

29. Which of the following is your *first* priority? To

    A give him oxygen and reassurance
    B prepare for an intravenous infusion
    C sit him up and loosen his clothing
    D take his observations and sit him up

30. Which of the following is an *immediate* complication of acute asthma:

    A cor pulmonale
    B emphysema
    C spontaneous pneumothorax
    D empyema

31. Which of the following *best* defines status asthmaticus:

    A a life threatening situation necessitating urgent treatment
    B a prolonged attack of asthma
    C a serious impairment of respiration
    D a condition which does not resolve within 4 hours

32. What is the priority of the nurse after subsidence of the initial attack. That

    A Simon has adequate rest and sleep
    B his respirations are recorded half-hourly
    C his airway is clear
    D his relatives are aware of the admission

29. C 34%

Sitting Simon upright and loosening any tight clothing, especially around the neck and waist, will be carried out first of all. His observations will then be taken, reassuring him during this time. An intravenous infusion may then be prepared if the doctor wishes to commence one. Oxygen may be given as it does reassure. Usually oxygen is given by nasal cannulae as these patients cannot generally tolerate oxygen masks on their faces.

30. C 40%

Pulmonary emphysema is distension of the alveoli with air. In asthma the air becomes trapped in the alveoli because of the constriction of the bronchioles, inspiration occurs but the patient cannot fully expire the air. A spontaneous pneumothorax occurs as a result of the rupturing of the visceral pleura and air entering the pleural space.
Empyema is pus within the lungs.
Cor pulmonale is heart disease following disease of the lungs which has caused strain on the right ventricle. The lung disease is usually chronic such as chronic bronchitis.
Hence C is an immediate complication, the others will take some time to arise.

31. A 28%

All of the options apply to status asthmaticus but A is the *best* definition. Asthma attacks should resolve or begin responding to treatment within 20 - 60 minutes. Continuation of the attacks result in status asthmaticus and these attacks exhaust the patient and prove life threatening.

32. D 54%

Options A, B and C will all be part of Simon's nursing care but it is important that his parents are informed of his admission as soon as possible. Simon's initial attack has subsided and he is conscious, therefore C will be achieved naturally by Simon and is not the nurse's priority.

Mark Green, aged 6 weeks, has been admitted with a diagnosis of congenital pyloric stenosis. His mother has accompanied him and is going to stay in the hospital.

33. Which of the following occurs in pyloric stenosis:

    A   inflammation of the pylorus
    B   thickening of the sphincter
    C   spasm of the duodenum
    D   incompetence of the muscle

34. Which of the following *must* be carried out prior to a Ramstedts operation:

    A   intravenous infusion to correct dehydration
    B   naso gastric tube in situ
    C   identity of baby checked
    D   skin and bowel preparation

35. Which of the following should be the priority following Mark's return from theatre:

    A   nurse him in a cubicle for the first 48 hours
    B   allow Mrs Green to care for Mark whenever possible
    C   allocate one nurse to care for Mark per shift
    D   tell parents not to worry on day of operation

36. Which of the following is most likely to be present when Mark is admitted:

    A   projectile vomiting
    B   abdominal distension
    C   diarrhoea and dehydration
    D   abdominal pain

Answers overleaf

33. **B**   66%

Thickening of the muscle blocks the outlet from the stomach, and the pyloric sphincter fails to relax normally to allow fluids from the stomach to pass into the duodenum. Thus stenosis (narrowing) of the pylorus occurs as a result of these changes.

34. **C**   44%

Although A, B and D may be part of the pre-operative care, C is absolutely essential in the interests of patient safety and must *always* be carried out.

35. **B**   32%

From the psychological aspect B is the priority as maternal bonding is important and it will also reassure and help Mrs Green to be present and involved in his care. There is no need to allocate one nurse specifically to look after Mark if his mother is present.

36. **A**   63%

The *most* likely presenting feature of pyloric stenosis in a 6 week old infant is projectile vomiting which is effortless. Because the pyloric sphincter is narrowed the stomach contents cannot pass into the duodenum, pressure within the stomach rises and effortless projectile vomiting results.

Miss Molly Hull has been admitted for investigations of weight loss and melaena. She consumes large doses of aspirin for migraine headaches and is withdrawn and difficult to communicate with.

37. Which of the following is a complication of aspirin over-indulgence:

   A diarrhoea
   B bleeding from the gums
   C gastric irritation
   D gastroenteritis

38. Which of the following is the best way to help develop a nurse/patient relationship:

   A try to find out if she has any domestic problems
   B talk about her hobbies and interests
   C tell her about yourself and observe her reactions
   D ask her if she has been dieting recently

39. Which of the following investigations will require a bowel preparation:

   A barium meal and swallow
   B gastroscopy and biopsy
   C sigmoidoscopy and barium study
   D rectal examination and proctoscopy

40. Miss Hull has passed a large melaena stool in the toilet. Which one of the following should the nurse do first:

   A call the doctor immediately
   B record pulse and blood pressure
   C bend her head forwards and ask her to take deep breaths
   D sit her in a wheelchair and return her to bed

Answers overleaf

37. C   85%

Aspirin causes gastric irritation and ulceration leading in severe cases to haematemesis or melaena. Large quantities may also lead to tinnitus.

38. B   57%

B is a means of establishing a relationship with the patient by showing an interest in her. A - as the patient is withdrawn she may feel the nurse is prying. She may not want to hear C, and D is a very pointed question which is not the best way to develop a relationship.

39. C   71%

Before both sigmoidoscopy and barium study it is essential that the colon is empty. If the bowel is not empty prior to barium enema faeces will distort the outline on the X-ray. A and B are investigations on the upper part of the alimentary tract, whilst the procedures in D both relate to the rectum and require no specific preparation.

40. D   56%

The priority will be her safe return to bed in case she collapses since she may have lost a large volume of blood. Once pulse and blood pressure have been recorded then the doctor will be notified.

Mr Organ, a retired businessman, is admitted to your ward with cirrhosis of the liver and severe haematemesis.

41. Which of the following is the reason for the bleeding:

    A oesophageal varices due to portal hypertension
    B a reduction in thrombocytes due to liver damage
    C a reduction in prothrombin due to liver damage
    D gastric venous engorgement due to portal hypertension

42. How may the discomfort resulting from the ascites of liver cirrhosis be minimized? By

    A pleural aspiration
    B prescribed sedation
    C paracentesis abdominis
    D prolonged anti-hypertensives

43. Why will Mr Organ complain of increasing pruritus? Due to the increased levels of

    A bile salts
    B bile pigments
    C cholesterol
    D sodium chloride

44. Why do some patients with cirrhosis develop mental confusion in the late stages? Because of

    A high blood potassium level
    B low blood urea level
    C high blood ammonia level
    D low blood glucose level

Answers overleaf

41. A 33%

Because Mr Organ has cirrhosis of the liver the congestion of the liver will affect the portal vein which drains blood into it. Pressure within the portal vein rises (hence the term portal hypertension) and is transmitted back to the organs of the alimentary canal system. Varicose veins develop in the oesophagus because of the high pressure within the veins, called oesophageal varices. If these varices rupture then bleeding occurs and the patient vomits the blood (haematemesis).

42. C 73%

Mr Organ will have excessive fluid in his abdominal cavity as a result of the portal hypertension which prevents venous reabsorption of tissue fluid. The ascites will cause abdominal distension and raised pressure on the diaphragm impairing breathing. Removal of the excess fluid by abdominal paracentesis will promote patient comfort. Cirrhosis of the liver cannot be cured, therefore treatment is palliative and aimed at relieving distressing symptoms whenever possible.

43. A 53%

Cirrhosis of the liver impairs normal liver function so the patient will gradually become jaundiced. As levels of bile salts rise and accumulate so the skin itches, whilst raised levels of bile pigment account for the yellow discolouration of skin and mucous membranes. (Pruritus means itching.)

44. C 23%

One of the functions of the liver is to convert excessive amino acids from protein digestion, firstly into ammonia, and then into urea for excretion by the kidneys. This process is incomplete when the liver is damaged, ammonia levels rise in the bloodstream and mental confusion results.

Ann James, aged 18 years, is admitted to your ward with a perforated appendix and is prepared for theatre.

45. Which of the following is the reason why Ann's stomach must be empty prior to a general anaesthetic? To

   A   reduce post-operative nausea
   B   reduce the production of hydrochloric acid
   C   stop peristalsis and paralytic ileus
   D   prevent inhalation of stomach contents

46. Which of the following is a secondary effect of post-operative pethidine? It

   A   diminishes nausea
   B   promotes diuresis
   C   encourages movement
   D   stimulates peristalsis

47. Which of the following is the main reason why nasogastric aspiration is performed post-operatively? To

   A   prevent paralytic ileus
   B   allow return of normal peristalsis
   C   reduce the flow of gastric juices
   D   ensure the patient is not nauseated

48. In which of the following stages of the nursing process would you determine whether Ann's post-operative care has been effective:

   A   evaluation
   B   planning
   C   implementation
   D   assessment

Answers overleaf

45. D   59%

Pre-operative fasting is an essential part of preparation for surgery because it reduces the risk of asphyxiation due to inhalation of stomach contents. Most patients are fasted for a minimum period of 6 hours in an attempt to ensure that the stomach is empty before the anaesthetic is administered. However, nursing research has highlighted the need to lengthen fasting times in very anxious patients as extreme anxiety can delay gastric emptying times.

46. C   39%

By relieving post-operative pain it is easier for the patient to move around the bed, thus the risk of complications from immobility are reduced.
The primary effect of pethidine is to relieve pain, hence C is a secondary effect.

47. D   34%

Paralytic ileus is likely after surgery for a perforated appendix therefore gastric juices will accumulate causing nausea and vomiting. Aspiration of a nasogastric tube will prevent this nausea.

48. A   61%

To "evaluate" the nursing care given means to decide how effective care has been. The patient's condition is compared to that anticipated by the nurse who planned the care initially and stated her aims of care at that time.

Miss Asquith, a 64 year old spinster who lives alone, has been unwell for some months with epigastric pain associated with meals, vomiting, anorexia and weight loss. A barium meal showed a possible neoplasm and an endoscopy was carried out.

49. Which form of endoscopy would be carried out:

    A enteroscopy
    B colonoscopy
    C oesophagoscopy
    D gastroscopy

50. Which of the following should be included as part of the pre-endoscopic management:

    A gastric lavage and insertion of a naso-gastric tube
    B naso gastric tube and aspiration
    C herculean preparation
    D preparation as for general anaesthetic

51. Following a barium meal Miss Asquith's potential problem is one of

    A constipation
    B anorexia
    C diarrhoea
    D vomiting

52. Which of the following is characteristic of a malignant tumour:

    A it is enclosed in a capsule and spreads rapidly
    B cells undergo active division and are enclosed in a capsule
    C it spreads rapidly and cells undergo active division
    D it can be recognised by culture with no infiltration

Answers overleaf

49. D 78%

After the barium meal has outlined the walls of the stomach Miss Asquith will also have a gastroscopy performed so that any suspect areas can be directly viewed via the gastroscope.

50. D 60%

As the doctor wishes to examine the stomach walls for abnormalities the patient must be fasted for 6 hours beforehand in an attempt to ensure that the stomach is empty, although a general anaesthetic is not necessary.

51. A 41%

After a barium meal the barium carries on through the alimentary tract and is excreted in the faeces. This may cause constipation therefore this is a potential (i.e. likely) problem for Miss Asquith.

52. C 77%

The other options are not characteristics of malignant tumours as they are not enclosed within a capsule and cannot be recognised by culture.

Silas Martin, a 45 year old bus driver, has a gastric ulcer for which he has received medical treatment. He is admitted to the ward in great distress having had a severe haematemesis.

53. Which of the following is a common site for gastric ulceration:

    A fundus
    B pylorus
    C greater curvature
    D lesser curvature

54. Which of the following is most likely to relieve the irritated gastric mucosa:

    A vomiting
    B eating
    C resting
    D alcohol

55. Which of the following is likely to be carried out initially on admission to the ward:

    A preparing Mr Martin for a barium meal
    B passing a naso-gastric tube and giving him milk orally
    C preparing him immediately for theatre
    D passing a naso-gastric tube and giving a blood transfusion

56. Which of the following would be most likely to indicate an improvement in Mr Martin's condition:

    A anxiousness to see his wife, and a slowing respiration rate
    B increasing movement in bed with an increasing respiration rate
    C anxiousness to get out of bed, and an increasing pulse rate
    D decreasing muscular strength with increasing peristaltic movement

Answers overleaf

53. D   27%

The common sites of ulceration are on the lesser curvature where trauma from the passage of food is likely to be greatest and repetitive. This trauma in the presence of gastric juice leads to ulceration especially when stimulation of gastric juice is enhanced; for example, by prolonged stressful situations. Mr Martin's driving job may be very stressful and exacerbate his ulcer.

54. A   25%

The presence of blood in the stomach causes considerable irritation to the mucous lining. The removal of this, along with irritating gastric juices by vomiting, will bring relief.

55. D   43%

Vomiting will empty the stomach but it is far better for the patient if this can be done without strain and stress. Aspiration of contents via a naso-gastric tube will do this. Because of the severe haematemesis he will also have a blood transfusion. These will be the initial actions on admission although theatre preparation may follow.

56. A   35%

This indicates that he is now able to give attention to things other than his intense personal suffering and a slowing respiration rate is a positive sign. Haemorrhage and shock give rise to a rapid respiration rate whilst restlessness can indicate further bleeding.

John, aged 18 months, has been admitted to the Paediatric Unit with a history of failure to thrive. A diagnosis of coeliac disease is made.

57. **Which of the following is a cause of coeliac disease:**

    A auto-immunity
    B infection
    C allergic reaction
    D heredity

58. **Coeliac disease is a condition in which there is**

    A oedema of the small bowel
    B ulceration of the large bowel
    C flattening of the villi
    D inflammation of the sigmoid colon

59. **A child with coeliac disease will be allowed to eat**

    A gluten-free bread
    B shredded wheat,
    C cornflakes,
    D a normal diet

60. **John's failure to thrive arises as a result of**

    A malabsorption of essential nutrients
    B too few pancreatic enzymes reaching the intestine
    C anorexia, vomiting and diarrhoea
    D inability to digest proteins and vitamins

Answers overleaf

Answers and explanations

57. C 60%

Coeliac disease is an allergic disorder. The allergen which stimulates the body's reaction is gluten, a substance found in wheat.

58. C 63%

Gradual flattening of the villi (finger-like projections of the small intestine) results in coeliac disease. This effectively reduces the surface area of small intestine available for absorption of nutrients.

59. A 11%

Because the child has an allergy to gluten, all wheat-based products must be avoided, this eliminates options B, C and D.

60. A 26%

Normally, the amino-acids, glucose, fatty acids and glycerol which are the end products of protein, carbohydrate and fat digestion, are absorbed into the bloodstream through the villi of the small intestine. Because the villi are flattened, malabsorption of essential nutrients takes place resulting in failure to thrive.

Mrs Harris, aged 40 years, is admitted with acute pancreatitis. She is obese and in a great deal of pain. This is Mrs Harris's first stay in hospital.

61. Which of the following enzymes is found in pancreatic juice:

   A pepsinogen
   B maltase
   C amylase
   D pepsin

62. What is a predisposing factor of pancreatitis? Excessive

   A carbohydrate intake
   B alcohol intake
   C hydrochloric acid secretion
   D dietary fibre

63. Which of the following actions will best reduce secretions from an acutely inflamed pancreas:

   A frequent aspiration of the stomach contents
   B administration of intravenous fluids
   C administration of antibiotics
   D frequent analgesia if needed

64. When planning for Mrs Harris's nursing care the nurse should

   A collect detailed information and identify the problems which are present
   B give the prescribed nursing care and record the patient's progress
   C decide upon nursing activities which will best provide individualised care
   D update the care plan as problems are overcome and priorities alter

Answers overleaf

61. C 63%

Pepsinogen is found in the gastric juice and maltase is found in the intestinal juice. Amylase, trypsinogen and lipase are the pancreatic enzymes.

62. B 53%

Many patients with acute pancreatitis have a history of excessive alcohol intake. Excessive secretion of hydrochloric acid could predispose peptic ulceration. Excessive carbohydrate intake for body requirements would eventually lead to obesity whilst excessive dietary fibre would simply be excreted and add bulk to the faeces.

63. A 53%

Aspiration of the stomach contents decreases pancreatic secretions. Intravenous fluids would maintain hydration, but alone would not decrease pancreatic secretions. Antibiotics and analgesics may be administered to control infection and pain respectively.

64. C 14%

Planning nursing care for a patient means prescribing the nursing care to overcome the identified problems/needs, thereby achieving individualised nursing care.
Assessing the patient's problems is achieved by collecting detailed information thereby enabling problems/needs to be identified.
Once the nursing care for the patient's problems has been prescribed, the care can be *implemented* by administering the care to the patient.
Evaluation of the patient's care plan is necessary in order to decide if the problem has been overcome and to update the care plan accordingly.

Mr Cosgrove is admitted to your ward for investigations of a suspected duodenal ulcer and magnesium trisilicate is prescribed. Following admission urgent surgery is necessary when perforation occurs.

65. Magnesium trisilicate is preferred to sodium bicarbonate because it is

   A   not absorbed into the blood stream
   B   a more effective antacid
   C   less likely to cause diarrhoea
   D   less likely to cause vomiting

66. For which of the following reasons is his magnesium trisilicate prescribed at regular times. In order to

   A   relax the pyloric sphincter
   B   inhibit gastric juice secretion
   C   promote healing of damaged mucosa
   D   form a protective coating

67. Which of the following *best* indicates that Mr Cosgrove's ulcer has perforated:

   A   dull abdominal pain
   B   an abnormal blood pressure
   C   severe haematemesis
   D   a rigid abdomen

68. Which of the following actions should you take first if he has not passed urine for 12 hours post-operatively:

   A   seek permission to perform catheterisation
   B   wheel the patient to the toilet and run the taps
   C   palpate the urinary bladder
   D   encourage fluids and record intake

Answers overleaf

65. A 24%

Sodium bicarbonate taken orally at frequent intervals can cause changes in the acidity/alkalinity of the bloodstream. Magnesium trisilicate is not absorbed in this way so is preferred as an antacid.

66. C 64%

By neutralising the acidity of the gastric juice which has eroded the mucosa of the alimentary tract, healing of the affected area will be enhanced.

67. D 27%

Perforation of a duodenal ulcer results initially in severe pain, hypotension and shock. As the ulcer has perforated, blood may enter the abdominal cavity and initiate peritonitis so haematemesis may not necessarily occur. Because of the pain, abdominal muscles may become rigid in order to guard the affected area and this, of the 4 alternatives given, *best* indicates perforation.

68. C 38%

Post-operatively Mr Cosgrove will be very ill making option B unrealistic. In the immediate post-operative period a paralytic ileus is likely and Mr Cosgrove will be having restricted oral intake so D is not feasible.
Catheterisation puts the patient at risk from ascending urinary tract infection and is not a first action.

Mrs Miles is an 88 year old lady who is about to be discharged home where she lives with her grand-daughter. Her only persistent problem is one of constipation.

69. Which of the following *best* describes constipation? When the patient

    A has not had a bowel action for 2 days
    B takes aperients regularly
    C has difficulty passing faeces
    D says she is constipated

70. Which of the following drugs may cause constipation:

    A codeine
    B cortisone
    C streptomycin
    D Digoxin

71. Bisacodyl suppositories cause the evacuation of faeces by

    A drawing water to the faeces
    B stimulating nerve endings in the rectum
    C lubricating the faeces
    D penetrating and softening the faeces

72. In an elderly patient frequent fluid faecal soiling is usually a sign of

    A ulcerative colitis
    B lack of sphincter control
    C gastroenteritis
    D faecal impaction

Answers overleaf

69. C   57%

A may be normal for the patient; some people have a bowel action 3 times a day, others twice a week.

B - careful use of aperients can prevent constipation.

C - the constipated patient has difficulty passing faeces and this can result in faecal impaction.

D - patients in hospital may claim to be constipated if they have not had a bowel movement every day, but this is not the best definition given.

70. A   62%

Codeine is a mild analgesic. It is used in cough mixtures, small doses are combined with aspirin and used as an analgesic and it is used as treatment for diarrhoea. It decreases peristalsis of the intestine and may cause constipation. B, C and D do not cause constipation.

71. B   24%

Bisacodyl suppositories act by stimulating the nerve endings in the large bowel and rectum. They do not lubricate, soften, or attract water to faeces.

72. D   44%

Ulcerative colitis is inflammation of the colon and rectum, causes diarrhoea, and affects people aged 20 - 40 years. Lack of sphincter control would result in faecal incontinence. Gastro-enteritis causes diarrhoea and may lead to incontinence. Faecal impaction in the elderly is usually the cause of frequent faecal fluid soiling, and such soiling should alert the nurse to this possibility.

Mr Peter Stevens, aged 76 years, is to undergo surgery for an enlarged prostate gland. He was admitted to hospital one week previously and has a urethral in situ.

73. Which of the following is the *most* common complication following catheterisation:

    A urethral stricture
    B muscle atonia
    C abdominal pain
    D ascending infection

74. Which of the following are essential aspects of Mr Stevens' pre-operative nursing care plan? To

    A promote mobilisation and encourage fluid intake
    B provide diversional therapy and physiotherapy
    C prevent insomnia and anxiety
    D perform a daily bedbath and oral toilet

75. What is the primary reason for recording urinary output in the immediate post-operative period? To

    A monitor renal function closely
    B detect clot retention of urine
    C monitor bladder capacity and tone
    D detect diminished urine production

76. Which of the following identifies the *most* likely problems after removal of Mr Stevens' catheter? A

    A risk of anuria and uraemia
    B tendency to develop haematuria
    C reluctance to drink adequate fluids
    D likelihood of urethral trauma

Answers overleaf

73. D 64%

In theory all options may result from catheterisation but the most common was requested. The risk of introducing organisms during catheterisation into the normally sterile bladder is great and once this happens the number of organisms increases and they may make their way, against the flow of urine, into the kidney pelvis. (i.e. Ascending from the bladder below to the kidneys above via the ureters.)

74. A 57%

Mr Stevens is to undergo quite major surgery for a man of his age and it is important to ensure that he is as fit as possible during the 7 days prior to operation. By encouraging movement and independence his recovery rate is enhanced and the risk of developing complications is much reduced. Similarly, if surgery is to be carried out, renal tract infection must be eliminated and a good urinary flow established pre-operatively. Options B, C and D may be desirable but A is essential.

75. B 70%

Post-operative bleeding may block the urethral catheter causing clot retention of urine. Adequate hydration, bladder washouts and accurate observation of urinary flow and colour should prevent the occurrence of this complication.

76. C 34%

The most likely potential problem is that Mr Stevens, on removal of his catheter, will be afraid that he will again develop urinary retention. Because of this he may be reluctant to drink thinking that by so doing he is helping the situation. In fact, the more he drinks the better it will be for him and nurses must encourage him to drink up to 3 litres of fluid daily.

Mr David Simpson, a 28 year old fitter, is admitted with right sided renal colic. He is unmarried and lives with his elderly parents.

77. Which of the following should be the nurses first priority when carrying out David's nursing care:

    A ensure that a urine specimen is obtained, sieved and tested
    B give the analgesia prescribed by the doctor
    C check that David's parents know of his admission
    D check David's temperature, pulse and blood pressure

78. Which of the following will initially assess David's renal function:

    A full blood count
    B micturating cystogram
    C abdominal X-ray
    D blood urea level

79. Which of the following actions should be taken immediately if David developed frank haematuria:

    A reassure him and tell him that this often happens
    B ask him to remain in bed and record his pulse half hourly
    C inform the doctor immediately of what has happened
    D tell him to drink plenty of fluids to prevent clot retention

80. Renal colic is described as a

    A constant ache in the loin radiating to the groin
    B sharp pain occurring in waves
    C severe constant pain related to micturition
    D persistent throbbing pain unrelieved by analgesia

Answers overleaf

77. **B   44%**

A is reasonable as urine must be tested on admission and sieved in this instance as renal colic is due to calculi - however it is not a first priority as you may have to wait some time for the urine specimen. B is the correct answer as David will be in a great deal of pain and distress and none of the other care procedures will be effective until this is minimised. C - as David lives with his parents they may be aware of his admission, if not they should be contacted if he wishes, however (as he is 28 years old) it is not the first priority. D - these observations are important, however they can be performed after the analgesia is given.

78. **D   55%**

A - a full blood count will not give any specific information about renal function. B - a micturating cystogram is usually performed to detect bladder abnormalities, e.g. reflux of urine into one or both ureters. It is therefore not specific to renal function. C - abdominal X-ray is not a test of renal function. D - Blood urea level is high if the kidneys cannot excrete urea therefore this gives information about renal function.

79. **C   68%**

A - David would need reassurance but it is not enough in this very serious situation and to tell him that this often happens is not really true and is too complacent when he requires urgent attention.
B - a pulse record should be kept and David should remain in bed but this will not help David immediately as he requires urgent attention.
C is correct as frank haematuria denotes haemorrhage and urgent surgical intervention may be required. D is wrong as until David has been assessed by the doctor he may need to be rushed to theatre and given an anaesthetic.

80. **B   78%**

A - the location of his pain is reasonable but the ache is typically spasmodic not constant. B is correct as it describes the nature of the pain which is thought to be due to increased peristaltic waves of the ureters attempting to overcome the obstruction caused by calculi. C - the pain is severe but spasmodic and is not usually related to micturition. D - analgesia is generally effective.

Donald Smith, aged 3 years, has within the last 4 weeks complained of a sore throat. He is admitted to hospital accompanied by both parents and a provisional diagnosis of acute glomerulonephritis is made.

81. Which of the following organisms would, in view of the diagnosis, be responsible for Donald's sore throat:

   A Streptococcus faecalis
   B Staphylococcus aureus
   C Haemolytic Streptococcus
   D Staphylococcus pyogenes

82. Which of the following would be found as an abnormal constituent of Donald's urine:

   A urea
   B creatinine
   C albumin
   D urochrome

83. Donald is prescribed 100 micrograms of a drug intramuscularly. The ampoule contained 0.5 milligrams in 2 millilitres. You should check and administer

   A 0.2 millilitres
   B 0.3 millilitres
   C 0.4 millilitres
   D 0.5 millilitres

84. When recording Donald's fluid balance chart, it is *most* important to

   A complete and check the chart totals before going off duty
   B measure the amount of fluid taken by mouth in 24 hours
   C measure and record fluid taken by mouth and lost by vomiting
   D complete the chart each time the patient has a drink, passes urine or vomits

Answers overleaf

Answers and explanations

81. C   41%

It is the haemolytic streptococcus toxins which cause bilateral inflammation of renal glomeruli - hence the term "glomerulonephritis". Streptococcus faecalis is an organism which is a cause of urinary tract infection.
Staphylococcus aureus is a pathogenic wound infecting organism.
Staphylococcus pyogenes is a pus producing organism.

82. C   56%

Albumin is an abnormal constituent and in the absence of disease is not filtered in the formation of urine as it is too large to pass into the tubule from the bloodstream.
Urochrome is a normal tissue pigment and urea and creatinine are normal constituents of urine.

83. C   26%

He is to be given 100 micrograms (0.1 mg).
500 micrograms (0.5 mg) in 2 millilitres is available.

Therefore $\frac{1}{5}$ of quantity available is to be given.

Therefore $\frac{1}{5} \times \frac{2}{1} = \frac{2}{5} = \frac{4}{10} = 0.4$ ml.

84. D   85%

A is not the answer because the time going off duty may not coincide with the end of a 24 hour period.
B and C do not consider all routes of fluid gain or loss.
D considers loss and intake and is therefore the answer and will ensure an accurate fluid chart at all times.

Mr Sidney Peters, aged 62 years, is in your ward with carcinoma of the bladder. He has been admitted for terminal nursing care.

85. Which of the following actions has priority when providing a reasonable quality of life? That

   A   skin and mouth hygiene is regularly carried out
   B   pain is assessed and controlled
   C   nourishing drinks are given as requested
   D   intake and output are closely monitored

86. Which of the following actions is the *most* important:

   A   administering his medication strictly on time
   B   using light weight bedclothes and incontinence pads
   C   allowing the family to be involved in his care
   D   requesting the doctor to prescribe sedation

87. Which of the following is likely to be a complication for Mr Peters:

   A   haematuria
   B   diarrhoea
   C   vomiting
   D   paraphimosis

88. When Mr Peters' death is imminent which of the following *must* the nurse ensure? That

   A   he is nursed in the side ward
   B   his bed is screened at all times
   C   he is not alone at the time of death
   D   relatives are present

Answers overleaf

85. B 74%

Control of pain is the most important aspect of care when caring for a patient with terminal carcinoma. This will enable the patient to be comfortable. The other distractors would be carried out routinely and do help, but when the patient is painfree he can be involved in his environment which will add to the quality of his remaining weeks of life.

86. C 63%

B and C may be needed, and whilst medication is essential, some flexibility of timing will be incorporated into his care to ensure adequate pain relief. However, in addition to unrestricted visiting, Mr Peter's family should be encouraged to be involved in his care - if they and the patient so wish. C is therefore the *most* important.

87. A 77%

The most likely complication of Mr Peter's carcinoma of the bladder is haematuria. (Paraphimosis is a painful retraction of the foreskin behind the glans penis.)

88. C 66%

No dying patient should be left alone to die, the mere fact that there is another person helps to lessen anxiety and fear. There is no need to isolate the patient or segregate him from other people. Relatives will be informed but may not be able to be present at all times, either for domestic or emotional reasons.

Mrs Green has just returned from theatre following stripping and ligation of varicose veins of her left leg. Her colour is good, pulse 84 and blood pressure 90/60 mmHg she is shivering, conscious but drowsy.

89. Which of the following nursing measures should the nurse perform:

    A raise the head of the bed, place her in the semi-prone position and report the pulse rate to sister

    B place her in a semi-recumbent position with a pillow under her left leg and report the shivering to sister

    C place an extra blanket next to her, put a cradle in the bed and report her blood pressure to sister

    D raise the foot of the bed, wash her face and hands and report her drowsiness to sister

90. Which of the following statements regarding Mrs Green's mobilisation is *most* appropriate? She should be

    A gradually mobilised to prevent the usual post-operative complications

    B walking very quickly after the operation so as to promote venous return

    C slowly mobilised to enable repair of the affected vein and suture line

    D allowed to sit only for the first two days post-operatively

91. Which of the following groups of factors predispose to the condition of varicose veins:

    A pregnancy, phlebitis and lack of exercise
    B faulty vein valves, standing and pregnancy
    C atheroma of vessels, obesity and poor footwear
    D deep vein thrombosis, standing and portal hypertension

92. Which of the following is the alternative form of treatment for varicose veins:

    A sclerosing injections
    B atrophic ointments
    C regular venograms
    D intensive physiotherapy

Answers overleaf

89. C 69%

The bed cradle is necessary because she has had an operation on her left leg and the blood pressure should be reported to sister as 90/60 mmHg, although not unusual following operation, is low. Care must be taken not to overheat Mrs Green, so only one extra blanket should be used although she is shivering.

90. B 19%

One large vein, often the long saphenous vein, has been stripped and ligated and venous return may not be very good. Therefore patients following this operation are mobilised as quickly as possible and encouraged to walk so that the leg muscles will improve venous return.

91. B 72%

Varicose veins occur in veins where valves have a weakness. Standing and pregnancy, although not causes, are predisposing factors because both tend to lead to pooling of venous blood. In pregnancy, hormones are released which help to relax smooth muscle and therefore there is a predisposition to varicose veins during pregnancy.

92. A 65%

Sclerosing injections are often successful and may be tried prior to operation. The drug used is a phenol preparation which scleroses ("hardens") the affected area of the vein and encourages alternative vessels to open up around it.

Mrs Jones, an obese middle-aged lady, is admitted to hospital suffering from iron deficiency anaemia.

93. Iron deficiency anaemia would be indicated by which of the following blood pictures:

   A small pale erythrocytes
   B large pale erythrocytes
   C large dark erythrocytes
   D small dark erythrocytes

94. The symptoms Mrs Jones would *most* likely complain of would be

   A pallor, tiredness,
   B weakness, palpitations
   C breathlessness, anorexia
   D anorexia, tiredness

95. If Mrs Jones' anaemia is so severe as to require a blood transfusion, the blood given would be

   A whole blood
   B plasma protein fraction
   C factor VIII concentrate
   D packed cells

96. A student nurse answers the telephone when Mrs Jones' daughters enquire about her condition. The learner should

   A refer to the Kardex report and give the answer
   B ask the senior nurse to speak to the daughters
   C ask the daughters to telephone later when the doctor will have seen their mother
   D tell them their mother is as comfortable as can be expected

Answers overleaf

93. **A** 28%

Iron gives the colour to red blood corpuscles so if iron is lacking the red corpuscles will be pale. As formation of the haemoglobin, using the iron, is one of the last stages in the formation of red cells, they are also very small, not large and immature.

94. **A** 21%

The most common symptoms of iron deficiency anaemia are pallor of skin and mucous membranes and tiredness caused by a lack of haemoglobin and resulting shortage of oxygen in the tissues.

95. **D** 59%

It is the quality not the quantity of Mrs Jones blood which is deficient therefore she already has the normal amount of blood circulating. To give whole blood would increase the risk of overloading the circulation therefore packed cells would be given.

96. **B** 57%

When answering telephone enquiries the nurse in charge should always be consulted to ensure that the most up to date information is given. "As comfortable as can be expected" is an unsatisfactory answer for it does little to allay relatives' anxiety.

Mr Haynes, aged 45 years, has severe hypertension and is admitted for observation and stabilisation of his blood pressure.

97. Which of the following is a hypotensive agent:

    A ferrous sulphate
    B methyldopa
    C aldosterone
    D praxilene

98. Which of the following is the *most* significant observation on admission:

    A blood pressure both standing and lying down
    B urinalysis in order to prevent renal involvement
    C anxiety state so that sedation may be ordered
    D apex beat to detect heart complications

99. Why is a standing blood pressure recorded when patients initially receive hypotensive agents? Because

    A there must be a difference of 30 mmHg between the systolic and diastolic pressures
    B the patient may suffer from postural hypotension when he moves suddenly
    C the recording obtained is generally lower than when sitting down
    D vasoconstriction occurs and ensures an increased cardiac output

100. Which of the follwing recordings is the *most* significant:

    A systolic of 130 mmHg
    B diastolic of 70 mmHg
    C systolic of 170 mmHg
    D diastolic of 100 mm Hg

Answers overleaf

97. B 69%

A hypotensive agent produces a low blood pressure (hypotension) or in the case of a patient with hypertension it reduces the blood pressure. Methyldopa is an anti-hypertensive or hypotensive agent.
Ferrous sulphate is an iron replacement.
Aldosterone is a salt retaining hormone.
Praxilene is a peripheral vaso-dilator.

98. A 61%

The most significant observation is the state of Mr Haynes' blood pressure, however his level of anxiety may aggravate and increase his blood pressure. Urinalysis will be conducted routinely. An apex beat may be done if there is an irregularity of his heart beat but this does not always occur with hypertension.

99. B 52%

A would not be achieved by recording a standing blood pressure and it is not necessary to maintain a difference of 30 mmHg.
B - hypotensive drugs decrease the blood pressure. If a patient moves from a lying or sitting position to a standing position suddenly, the blood pressure may not immediately be maintained and the patient will feel dizzy. Therefore a standing blood pressure is recorded to prevent hypotensive drugs decreasing the blood pressure excessively.
C - the recording is generally lower when the patient stands up.
D is not the reason for recording a standing blood pressure although vasoconstriction must occur on standing up to maintain an adequate cerebral blood flow.

100. D 59%

The systolic blood pressure is the force exerted when the heart pumps blood around the body. The average systolic pressure is 120 mmHg however this may increase with age at a rate of 10 mm per 10 years from the age of twenty, so a systolic pressure of 140 mm is acceptable for a 40 year old. However the diastolic pressure is the pressure of the heart at rest, on average, 70 mm. An increase in the diastolic pressure means that the heart is under considerable strain even at rest therefore D is correct.

Mrs Adams, a 50 year old lady, has been admitted to hospital for investigation and treatment of vitamin B_{12} deficiency anaemia.

101. Which of the following best describes the result of the anaemia:

A enlargement of the liver and spleen
B a fall in the circulatory volume of blood
C a reduction in the oxygen carrying capacity of blood
D a reduction in the number of red cells

102. When Mrs Adams is given a blood transfusion, which of the following would cause you *most* concern:

A nausea and loss of appetite
B headache and lethargy
C cold feeling in the vein of the arm
D dyspnoea and tachycardia

103. Which of the following antigens (agglutinogens) are found in group AB blood:

A A only
B B only
C A and B
D no antigens at all

104. Which of the following causes haematuria to occur during a blood transfusion:

A breakdown of the red cells
B allergic reaction
C retention of urine
D overloading of the circulation

101. C   34%

Anaemia *always* results in reduction of the oxygen carrying capacity of blood either because of a reduction in quantity or quality of the red cells.

Anaemia may result in slight enlargement of the spleen in haemolytic anaemia due to an increased rate of breakdown of red cells.

Anaemia is not due to loss of blood caused by acute or chronic haemorrhage in Mrs Adams case.

102. D   79%

D would cause most concern as dyspnoea and an increased pulse rate indicate a rise in blood volume resulting in acute pulmonary oedema which is a medical emergency.

Nausea, loss of appetite and headache are not life threatening and may or may not be connected with the anaemia.

A cold feeling may be experienced in the vein of the arm if the blood transfused is not at the correct temperature.

103. C   56%

Agglutinogen A is found in blood group A.

Agglutinogen B is found in blood group B.

Agglutinogens A and B are found in blood group AB.

Group O has no agglutinogens.

The blood group is named according to the agglutinogens present on the red blood cell.

104. A   12%

Agglutination (clumping together of red cells) can occur in transfused blood due to incompatibility. In the kidney this causes pain in the loin and haematuria. The haematuria arises due to the haemolysis (breakdown) of the red cells and the release of haemoglobin which passes to the renal tubules.

An allergic reaction would not cause haematuria but may cause for example, skin rash.

Retention of urine would not occur as there would be no blockage to the outflow of urine. Overloading of the circulation would cause acute dyspnoea and rise in pulse rate, cough and tightness in the chest but not haematuria.

Mr James is brought into casualty with severe chest pain, radiating down his left arm. While preparing for the doctor's examination you are unable to detect a carotid pulse. He is now in a collapsed state with dilated pupils and absence of respirations.

105. Which of the following should be your priority? To

    A go for help and fetch a doctor
    B draw the curtains and telephone "cardiac arrest"
    C commence artificial resuscitation
    D lie Mr James flat and protect his airway

106. Which of the following groups of drugs may be given during resuscitation:

    A adrenaline, lignocaine, frusemide
    B lignocaine, sodium bicarbonate, adrenaline
    C digoxin, adrenaline, sodium bicarbonate
    D morphine, aminophylline, frusemide

107. Before applying defibrillation to Mr James it must be observed that

    A Mr James is not wearing anything metal
    B there is no metal in the vicinity
    C no-one is touching Mr James or the trolley
    D no-one is in the vicinity of Mr James

108. Once Mr James is conscious and has recovered from the resuscitation you should position him

    A flat with the foot of the bed elevated
    B semi-recumbent with head supported
    C semi-prone, protecting his airway
    D prone with one pillow

Answers overleaf

105. C   49%

The patient has arrested and it is essential to commence artificial resuscitation as soon as possible.

The other actions will also be completed in the cardiac arrest procedure; call for help but stay with the patient - someone else can summon the doctor. When summoned, someone else will draw the curtains and telephone. Lie Mr James flat but you need to commence resuscitation as well as protecting the airway.

106. B   59%

Some of these drugs may be given during a cardiac arrest situation although some are to stabilise and improve the patient's condition *after* the arrest e.g. Digoxin will slow, steady and strengthen the heart beat.

Frusemide is a diuretic which aids in reducing circulatory overload. The question asked which drugs are given during the arrest, so B is correct. Sodium bicarbonate is given in every arrest situation to correct the acidosis of the body. Adrenaline may be given directly into the heart or intravenously to stimulate the heart into action and Lignocaine is given to calm the heart muscle and produce regular controlled heart rhythm.

107. C   75%

Defibrillation is the passage of an electrical current to the patient to stimulate the heart into normal action. No one should touch Mr James, his trolley or anything attached to him, or they will likewise receive the electrical current and this may cause a normal heart action to become abnormal. Therefore, before the electrical impulse is conducted, the doctor must ask everyone not to touch the patient or trolley.

108. B   73%

Following recovery from resuscitation, conscious patients are usually placed in a semi-recumbent position ensuring that the head is comfortable. If Mr James were not fully recovered, or unconscious, then a different position would be used in order to facilitate recovery and protect the patient.

Mrs Mary Gooch, a 64 year old lady, is brought into the medical ward following a domiciliary visit. She looks very pale, her sclera are slightly yellow, she is breathless, lethargic and has some ankle oedema. Her Hb is 3.4 grammes/per decilitre (3.4 g/dl).

109. Which of the following statements is appropriate regarding the likelihood of Mrs Gooch developing decubitus ulcers:

    A the risk is slight as she is breathless but not paralysed or incontinent
    B she will not be totally confined to bed therefore the risk is reduced
    C generalised tissue anoxia and lethargy constitute a high risk
    D her age and likely disorientation associated with admission is relevant

110. Which of the following groups of nursing observations is *most* likely to help the doctor make his/her diagnosis:

    A temperature, urinalysis and respiratory rate
    B colour of stool, pulse and state of tongue
    C degree of pallor, weight and blood pressure
    D urine output, function of limbs and dietary habits

111. Mrs Gooch's plan of care provides for the nursing staff to help with all daily living activities. The reason for this is to

    A prevent the complication of heart failure
    B monitor her exercise tolerance
    C prevent psychological disturbance and depression
    D re-establish a normal pattern of self care

112. Following diagnosis, injections of Neo-Cytamen are prescribed. The reason for this is to

    A replace the depleted iron stores in the body
    B stimulate the bone marrow to replace red corpuscles
    C provide the missing factor necessary for red corpuscle maturation
    D enhance absorption of the extrinsic factor from the gut

Answers overleaf

109. C   58%

Mrs Gooch is seriously anaemic with a haemoglobin of only 3.4 g/dl and therefore the tissues are going to be starved of oxygen. She is lethargic, and this will constitute a high risk as far as the production of pressure sores is concerned especially as bed rest will be ordered until her haemoglobin level rises.

110. B   37%

The nursing observations which are most likely to help the doctor to make a diagnosis are those which would assist in determining the type of anaemia. B is correct as the colour of the stool will show if there is any frank bleeding into the stool or altered blood in the stool which may help to indicate gastro-intestinal bleeding. The pulse is important because again this may be an indication of internal haemorrhage. The state of the mouth and tongue are important because glossitis is not an uncommon situation, particularly in pernicious anaemia.

111. A   16%

This patient is severely affected, her heart is under a great deal of strain and if she continues to attempt to carry out basic care for herself then she is going to become extremely breathless and her heart will be embarrassed further. Therefore the nursing staff will help her with all her daily living activities in order to prevent the complication of heart failure.

112. C   34%

Neo-Cytamen is a preparation of vitamin B_{12} and this is given to provide the missing factor necessary for red corpuscle maturation. As she has a vitamin B_{12} deficiency anaemia her red cells will be large and immature and will break up much more quickly. The factor is replaced by injections of the drug and then the red corpuscles can mature normally.

Mr Roland Smith, a bank manager, is undergoing tests to discover the cause of his hypertension which he has suffered now for some months. He is a 41 year old widower with 2 children aged 10 years and 8 years. Their aunt, who is a health visitor in London, has taken annual leave to care for them whilst Mr Smith is in hospital.

113. Which of the following groups of symptoms is Mr Smith likely to have suffered:

    A   chest pain and frequency of micturition
    B   giddiness and headache
    C   tremor and insomnia
    D   oliguria and intermittent claudication

114. Which of the following is the reason for investigations of renal function:

    A   function of all the body systems is carried out to discover cause of hypertension
    B   hypertension causes renal damage and the extent of this aids diagnosis
    C   hypertension is sometimes secondary to conditions affecting the renal system
    D   hypotensive drugs may damage the kidneys, therefore their function is determined prior to treatment

115. Which of the following is the *most* important reason for the ward sister ensuring that Mr Smith's tests are performed on schedule? Any delay will cause

    A   serious domestic problems
    B   financial hardship
    C   physical deterioration
    D   business difficulties

116. Which of the following organisations is specifically concerned with helping single parent families:

    A   Mencap
    B   Gingerbread
    C   Child guidance
    D   Samaritans

Answers overleaf

113. B   80%

Signs and symptoms of hypertension are often very slight and the more serious problems that ensue are complications of the hypertension, so if Mr Smith had suffered any signs and symptoms they are likely to be headache and occasional giddiness.

114. C   53%

Mr Smith is being investigated to discover the cause of his hypertension, and conditions affecting the renal system sometimes lead to hypertension e.g. stag horn calculus, renal tumours, stenosis of the renal arteries.

If the kidneys are not working correctly then salt and water may be retained in the body and renin may be produced from the kidneys which raises the blood pressure. Hence tests of renal function will identify renal cause of the raised blood pressure.

115. A   41%

Mr Smith has managed to get the children's aunt, who is herself a health visitor in London and presumably in full time employment, to take annual leave to care for the children. The children are only 10 and 8 years of age and as he needed to make these arrangements one would imagine that a lengthened stay in hospital could create very serious domestic problems for him as he may have no one else to care for his children.

B and D are unlikely because of the nature of his job and C could occur but the delay would need to be quite lengthy.

116. B   85%

The Gingerbread organisation is the only one of the four mentioned which specifically helps one parent families although certainly A, C and D could help them in addition to other members of society.

Heather Wright, aged 6 years, has been having repeated sore throats causing her to lose a lot of time at school. She is admitted to the E.N.T. ward for a tonsillectomy.

117. Heather's parents were encouraged to visit whenever possible primarily to ensure they could

   A be less anxious about her
   B maintain parental control
   C prevent regression
   D give support and care

118. Which of the following would *best* indicate that Heather was bleeding after her operation:

   A sweating, tachycardia, hyperventilation
   B tachycardia, restlessness, swallowing
   C swallowing, sweating, anxiety
   D hyperventilation, restlessness, vomiting

119. Immediately post-operatively it is *most* important to ensure that

   A she can swallow fluids easily
   B her analgesia is given as prescribed
   C she is not swallowing excessively
   D her temperature, pulse and respirations are normal

120. The doctor has prescribed analgesia, 0.06 of a millilitre per year of age. How much solution should you draw up in the syringe:

   A 3.6 mls
   B 3.06 mls
   C 0.36 ml
   D 0.366 ml

Answers overleaf

117. **D**   78%

The primary reason for encouraging Heather's parents to visit whenever possible is so that they can help with her nursing care and give support to their daughter during a worrying time. Options A, B and C may also result from an open visiting policy but will arise because D is being carried out.

118. **B**   68%

If Heather is bleeding from the tonsil bed she is likely to swallow the blood as it trickles down her throat, become restless as a result of the blood loss and have an increased heart rate as the heart attempts to maintain an adequate blood supply to all body organs. Of the alternatives given those in B would best indicate haemorrhage.

119. **C**   57%

Excessive swallowing is usually the first sign of bleeding before there is alteration in baseline recordings. Heather will only take fluids when she is fully conscious, not immediately post-operatively and analgesia may not be needed immediately.

120. **C**   80%

0.06 ml per year of age.
Heather is 6 years of age and therefore requires 0.06 x 6 = 0.36 ml.

Mr Robert Jones is admitted for a sub-mucous resection of the nasal septum.

121. Which of the following must Mr Jones be told about regarding his post-operative state:

    A he must not remove the nasal pack
    B he will breathe normally within 24 hours
    C 4 hourly nose blowing is important
    D there will be an external wound

122. Why is blood pressure recorded and urinalysis carried out pre-operatively? In order to

    A check renal function
    B carry out baseline recordings
    C screen for undiagnosed diseases
    D detect early heart failure

123. How will post-operative haematoma formation be prevented? By

    A frequent nose blowing and inhalations
    B keeping a nasal pack in position
    C 4 hourly nose drops causing vasoconstriction
    D ice compresses and pressure externally

124. Which of the following will be carried out to facilitate reduction of the swelling of the mucous membranes:

    A Naseptin cream 4 hourly
    B ice packs on the bridge of the nose
    C antihistamine cream for nose
    D steam inhalations 4 hourly

121. **A   84%**

Nasal packs are inserted following a sub-mucous resection of the nasal septum to prevent a haematoma from forming between the mucous membranes where the septum has been removed.
B and D are incorrect and nose blowing will be positively discouraged as a nasal pack is in situ.

122. **C   38%**

All patients should have their urine tested and blood pressure recorded pre-operatively in order to rule out diabetes and hypertension of which the patient has been unaware.

123. **B   32%**

Haematoma forming between the mucous membranes at the septum will prevent healing and may lead to infection so this must be prevented by constant pressure from a nasal pack.

124. **D   5%**

Steam inhalations help to reduce swelling of the mucous membranes post-operatively as the warmth from the steam encourages blood flow which in turn aids reabsorption of excessive tissue fluid.

Penny is an intelligent extrovert 12 year old, the only child of middle aged parents. Whilst attending a history lesson at school she had a grand mal epileptic fit. Penny is admitted to the ward fully conscious, accompanied by her very anxious and rather overpowering mother.

125. Which of the following should be the policy regarding the degree of mobility that Penny is allowed in hospital:

    A give a prescribed sedative and maintain strict bed rest for 24 hours

    B allow her to sit quietly by her bed and ring for a nurse if she wishes to go to the toilet

    C restrict her movements to walking around her bed and going to the toilet

    D allow her to be up and around but ensure you know her whereabouts

126. Which of the following should be your priority action when Penny has a further grand mal fit whilst watching television in the dayroom:

    A lie her on the floor, clear all furniture from the immediate vicinity

    B turn her head to one side to drain secretions, place a wooden spatula between her teeth

    C lie her semi-prone on the floor, ask another nurse to fetch an oxygen cylinder

    D turn her head to one side to drain secretions, ask other patients to leave the day-room

127. Which of the following correctly lists in order some of the stages of an epileptic fit:

    A tonic, clonic, automatism, coma

    B aura, clonic, tonic, sleep

    C clonic, tonic, sleep, automatism

    D aura, tonic, clonic, sleep

128. Which of the following may Penny initially find the most difficult:

    A telling her relatives about her condition

    B returning to school and facing her friends

    C being reliant on medication to stabilise her epilepsy

    D the thought of being overprotected by her mother

Answers overleaf

125.

D 61%

Penny is in hospital for investigation and observation and this can be carried out quite adequately as long as you know where she is. Bed rest would not be required as Penny is fully conscious. It is also unlikely that a sedative would be prescribed as this may mask important signs and symptoms which need to be detected early.

The restrictions in B and C are unnecessary and may make her unhappy.

126. A 69%

A is correct as it maintains patient safety by prevention of further injury.

B is unsafe - if you turn her head it will probably only jerk back again and putting anything between the teeth is usually impossible and may damage the teeth.

Oxygen is not useful - the reason for cyanosis in fitting is the rigidity of the respiratory muscles.

D - neither of these actions is particularly useful to your patient.

127. D 64%

The classic stages of an epileptic fit are:

1. Aura - warning of fit.
2. Tonic phase - rigidity of muscle groups.
3. Clonic phase - alternate rigidity and relaxation.
4. Coma and sleep - unconsciousness lessening gradually in depth.
5. Automatism (very rare occurrence when patient may appear to be normal but have no real control over actions).

128. B 64%

Since the original fit occurred at school, Penny will have to face her schoolmates and explain the situation to them herself. It is very likely that her parents will tell the relatives so this is unlikely to be difficult for her.

As the usual medication is taken orally this is not likely to be a problem.

It is difficult to judge what option D may mean to her - but most children accept their parents. It is outsiders who consider over protectiveness a problem and initially Penny may be glad of it.

Mr Brockbank, 65 years old, has a laryngeal carcinoma causing obstruction to his respiration. He wishes to be nursed at home during his last months. A palliative tracheostomy is to be performed.

129. Suction should be applied post-operatively

   A   on entry of the catheter
   B   using a 60 ml syringe and catheter
   C   as the catheter is withdrawn
   D   2 hourly using an aseptic technique

130. Immediately post-operatively the equipment close to hand should include

   A   artery forceps
   B   laryngoscope
   C   tracheal dilators
   D   Michel clip removers

131. If the disposable tracheostomy tube becomes blocked during the first few hours post-operatively, the nurse should first

   A   telephone for the doctor to change the tube
   B   take out the tube and replace with a new one
   C   remove the tube and maintain patency of the opening
   D   continue to apply suction until the blockage is cleared

132. If a silver tracheostomy tube is to be taken home his wife should be taught that the tube

   A   should only be touched by the district nurse
   B   has a lining which can be removed for cleaning
   C   never becomes obstructed
   D   can only be changed by a doctor

129. C 83%

Suction should only be applied upon withdrawal of the catheter so as to avoid damage to the tracheal lining. Timing cannot be too specific, it must always be performed when necessary according to the patient's condition.

130. C 73%

If the tracheostomy tube becomes dislodged or blocked it must be removed and tracheal dilators inserted immediately to keep the stoma open. Urgent medical help must then be summoned.

131. C 45%

Remove the tube and insert the tracheal dilators and send for help. The surgeon will re-insert a new tracheostomy tube as this is difficult during the first few post-operative hours.

132. B 66%

The silver Negus tube has 3 parts: an introducer, a lining tube, and an external tube. In the home the lining is removed for cleaning and replaced, after sterilisation by boiling.

Stephen Collinson, a 16 year old school boy, is admitted in a hyperglycaemic (diabetic) coma. He lives with his parents and 3 younger brothers in a three bedroomed bungalow. The whole family has recently had an attack of influenza.

133. Which of the following is the first priority in Stephen's management on admission:

   A record baseline observations
   B maintain a clear airway
   C obtain and test a urine specimen
   D identify nursing problems

134. Which of the following statements *best* describes the action of insulin? It

   A allows glucose to enter the cells
   B converts glycogen back to glucose
   C raises the level of glucose in the plasma
   D prevents abnormal metabolism of fat

135. What is the reason for Stephen's treatment with fluids and insulin? It is because he

   A is prone to infection and has a low blood glucose level
   B has ketosis, polyuria and pyrexia
   C is unconscious and has acidosis
   D has a high blood glucose level and dehydration

136. When Stephen is ready for discharge he needs to take a controlled amount of carbohydrate over a 24 hour period. The primary reason for this is

   A to prevent the likelihood of glycosuria
   B to prevent the occurrence of hypoglycaemia
   C that insulin and carbohydrate are calculated together
   D that carbohydrate intake is calculated to maintain normal body weight

Answers overleaf
67

133. B   80%

Stephen is in a diabetic coma therefore he is unconscious and the priority in management must be maintenance of a clear airway. A, C and D will be carried out, but A must come first.

134. A   46%

Option A most accurately describes the action of insulin, this is the way in which it facilitates the body's use of glucose. B and C are incorrect and D is not a direct mechanism, although complete fat metabolism only occurs when blood sugar level is normal.

135. D   73%

The action of insulin is to lower the blood glucose level, whilst intravenous fluids will correct dehydration. This is present in hyperglycaemic patients because of the kidneys' attempts to excrete as much of the excess glucose as possible.

136. C   50%

The amount of carbohydrate in the diet and the amount of insulin prescribed by the doctor are worked out in combination. This is in order to maintain as normal a blood glucose level as possible and to prevent ketosis which occurs when fat is incompletely metabolised.

Mrs Dickens is admitted to your ward with a suspected overactive thyroid gland.

137. Which of the following groups are representative of the clinical features which may be present:

   A   sweating, tachycardia, increased appetite
   B   exophthalmos, menorrhagia, sweating
   C   tremor, lethargy, tachycardia
   D   exophthalmos, oliguria, increased appetite

138. Cardiac involvement may result in

   A   coupled beats
   B   bradycardia and arrhythmia
   C   hypotension and angina
   D   ventricular hypertrophy

139. Which of the following is a specific complication which may occur post-operatively:

   A   hypercapnoea
   B   hypernatraemia
   C   hypocalcaemia
   D   hypovolaemia

140. Which of the following is the primary reason for using clips to unite the wound? Because they

   A   are easier to remove in an emergency
   B   do not have to stay in as long as sutures
   C   leave a neater scar line
   D   are more comfortable for the patient

137. A   47%

Menorrhagia, lethargy and oliguria are not characteristics of thyrotoxicosis, thus options B, C and D are incorrect.
Sweating, tachycardia, increased appetite and tremor will be found when a patient has an overactive thyroid gland due to the increased metabolic rate. Exopthalmos (protruding eyes) is also present.

138. D   36%

Because of the prolonged tachycardia it is possible for a patient's left ventricle to enlarge (hypertrophy) in an attempt to maintain cardiac output. If the thyrotoxicosis is untreated heart failure may eventually occur.

139. C   58%

If the parathyroid tissue is also removed during the partial thyroidectomy the serum calcium levels will fall due to lack of parathormone resulting in tetany. Any muscle spasm must be reported immediately.

140. C   38%

The primary reason for using clips to unite the wound is that a neat scar line results. This is an important factor when you consider the site of this scar, particularly so for female patients.

Angela Green has just returned from theatre having undergone a partial thyroidectomy.

141. Why is Angela prescribed potassium iodide pre-operatively? Because it reduces

  A thyroxine levels
  B the risk of haemorrhage
  C serum calcium levels
  D gland size

142. Which of the following is a specific post-operative complication:

  A laryngeal nerve damage
  B wound infection
  C deep vein thrombosis
  D chest infection

143. Which of the following is the reason why hyoscine (scopolamine) and atropine are given as premedication? Because primarily they

  A cause amnesia
  B prevent vomiting
  C minimise secretions
  D prolong the effect of anaesthesia

144. Reactionary haemorrhage occurs usually

  A at the time of the operation
  B whilst the patient is in the recovery room
  C between 1 and 24 hours post-operatively
  D up to 10 days post-operatively

Answers overleaf

141.   B   43%

The thyroid gland takes up iodine from the blood stream in order to manufacture thyroxine, therefore it is a very vascular organ, liable to bleed easily during surgery. By giving potassium iodide pre-operatively the gland's supply of iodine is increased, it becomes firmer and less vascular thus lowering the risk of haemorrhage.

142.   A   59%

Options B, C and D are all post-operative complications but each may arise after any type of surgery. Laryngeal nerve damage can occur during partial thyroidectomy because it is situated near to the gland and so of the 4 alternatives it is the only *specific* complication.

143.   C   71%

Scopolamine and atropine have very similar effects - they diminish the amount of gastric juice and saliva produced as well as slowing down peristalsis. This is their primary action, although vomiting may be reduced as a result.

144.   C   68%

Primary haemorrhage occurs at the time of injury.
Reactionary haemorrhage is likely during the first 24 hours post-operatively as the blood pressure rises.
Secondary haemorrhage results from infection of the operation site and so occurs between 7 and 10 days post-operatively.

Mrs Adams, aged 40 years, has recently been diagnosed as having rheumatoid arthritis and has been prescribed Plaster of Paris back splints for her hands and a course of steroid drugs.

145. Which of the following is the best definition of rheumatoid arthritis:

A an inflammatory disease of the small joints
B an inflammatory condition of joints associated with weightbearing
C a disease of all joints causing pain, swelling and deformity
D a disease of large joints caused by previous infection

146. Which of the following instructions will be given to Mrs Adams? To apply the splints

A just during daytime to prevent injuring her joints
B when her hands are painful and need resting
C for most of the 24 hours to maintain natural position
D before attending physiotherapy to rest the joints

147. Which is the *most* appropriate response if Mrs Adams expresses concern about the likelihood of becoming severely disabled:

A the nurse is not able to predict a prognosis but the doctor will give her information
B many people are handicapped by the disease but she may not necessarily be one of them
C that nursing care and rehabilitation will be carefully planned to prevent disability
D if disabilities should arise her care and treatment will be planned to help her overcome them

148. Mrs Adams' main anxiety is her changing facial features and excessive facial hair. It is important to ensure that she

A understands the effects of steroid drugs and achieves a high standard of dress and appearance
B understands the effects of steroid drugs and gradually looses weight
C gradually loses weight and receives advice regarding hair removal
D reduces steroids rapidly and has facial hair removed

Answers overleaf

145. **A   16%**

Rheumatoid arthritis is an inflammatory disease of synovial joints; the cause is unknown but auto-immunity is thought to play a part. Abnormal immunoglobulins (antibodies) are found in the blood of sufferers - this is known as the rheumatoid factor. Not all joints are affected and weightbearing is not a factor. Similarly there is no connection with previous infections.

146. **C   52%**

Back splints are fitted to hold the inflamed joints in a natural position so as to reduce deformity and pain. They should be worn day and night except for periods of physiotherapy until the acute inflammatory phase of the disease is over.

147. **D   43%**

The prognosis of the condition is difficult to assess in the early stages.
A is not a satisfactory answer as the nurse is not meeting the patient's immediate need for an answer. B is not a helpful statement. C - the prevention of disability cannot be assured by management. D is the best answer in the circumstances as the patient is assured that she will not be left to cope alone should disability arise.

148. **A   24%**

The changes are due to steroid therapy. It is important that the patient understands this and that she continues to take an interest in herself.
Dieting may not be effective under these circumstances as it will not stop the changing of her features. If steroid therapy is reduced suddenly Mrs Adams may collapse, so option D is incorrect.

Mrs Cooke, aged 58 years, has been admitted to your ward with a diagnosis of rheumatoid arthritis. One week following admission Mrs Cooke had a severe haematemesis.

149. Which of the following is the *most* likely cause of Mrs Cooke's haematemesis? Because she

   A   is worried and anxious
   B   is receiving indomethacin capsules
   C   has achlorhydria
   D   has had dyspepsia for years

150. Which of Mrs Cooke's joints will *first* be affected by rheumatoid arthritis? Her

   A   spine
   B   hips and knees
   C   hands and fingers
   D   shoulders

151. The main aim of Mrs Cooke's plan of care is to

   A   re-establish independence
   B   maintain her dignity
   C   preserve her personal hygiene
   D   allay her fears by communication

152. In order to increase Mrs Cooke's motivation towards her goals of care which of the following would be *most* important? The nurse should

   A   always reward whether goal is achieved or not
   B   only reward when perfection is finally achieved
   C   aim to over-motivate rather than under-motivate
   D   make sure her goals are achievable

Answers overleaf

149. B   71%

Indomethacin capsules are recommended to be taken with milk since a side effect of the drug is peptic ulceration. Haematemesis would indicate peptic ulceration.
Although A and D could possibly indirectly be associated with haematemesis they would not be the *most* likely cause. C is an unassociated factor.

150. C   73%

The metacarpophalangeal joints are the joints usually affected first. Although other joints become involved later, the disease first starts in the hands and feet.

151. A   66%

The progression of rheumatoid arthritis varies greatly from patient to patient, but since the disease is marked by periods of remission and exacerbation the main aim of care will be to re-establish independence.
B, C and D will also be aims of care but the question asks for the *main* aim.

152. D   60%

In order to increase motivation for any patient with a progressive disease, goals of care must be both realistic and achievable so that the patient does not feel a sense of failure.
A, B and C would not serve to actually increase the patient's motivation in any way.

Miss Plant is 59 years old and has severe osteoarthrosis of the hip joint. She is admitted for a Charnley operation.

153. **Which of the following is a correct statement:**

    A   this is a palliative measure since the osteoarthrosis will re-occur in the same hip

    B   full recovery of joint movement is possible after the operation

    C   ambulation is possible after the operation but Miss Plant will need to refrain from strenuous exercise

    D   the degree of recovery of movement will depend on the severity of the osteoarthrosis before the operation

154. **Osteoarthrosis is caused by which of the following:**

    A   degeneration of the joint due to articulation

    B   infection of the synovial membrane of the joint

    C   infection and erosion of the long bone

    D   bone chip formation and narrowing of the joint space

155. **Which of the following is the correct position of the hip following a Charnley operation:**

    A   adducted using a Charnley mattress to encourage lateral rotation

    B   abducted to discourage rotation and dislocation

    C   immobilised with Hamilton Russell traction

    D   adducted and immobilised with traction for 48 hours

156. **Which of the following would be the safest way to prevent pressure sore development in the immediate post-operative period:**

    A   turn the patient gently from side to side 2 hourly

    B   sit the patient out of bed as soon as possible and mobilise gently

    C   with another nurse lift the patient's sacrum from the bed every 2 hours

    D   use a sheepskin and encourage Miss Plant to use the monkey pole to change position.

Answers overleaf

153. **B** 38%

Once healing has taken place, with effective rehabilitation and physiotherapy, full recovery of joint movement is possible. Only in a few cases would the patient have the potential to achieve less after the operation than before.

154. **A** 43%

Osteoarthrosis is a degenerative disorder which essentially affects the weightbearing joints such as the hips and knees. The articulation (movement) aggravates the situation as the articular cartilage protecting the bone ends of the joints becomes cracked and thinned.

155. **B** 41%

After hip replacement surgery it is important to prevent dislocation by keeping the prosthesis firmly in place in the hip socket. This is best achieved by abducting (moving away from the body) the leg at an angle of 45 degrees and keeping it in this position by using a foam wedge.

156. **C** 13%

The other 3 options will all cause dislocation of the hip therefore C is the correct answer.

Ray Lancaster, aged 21 years, has had a torn cartilage in his knee for some months. It causes pain, locking of the joint and swelling and he has been advised to have the cartilage removed surgically.

157. The operation to remove a cartilage from the knee is called

    A patellectomy
    B mastoidectomy
    C synovectomy
    D meniscectomy

158. Which of the following is the *most* important aspect of Mr Lancaster's pre-operative nursing preparation:

    A knee exercises four times daily
    B group and cross-match 2 units of blood
    C skin preparation to reduce the risk of infection
    D anticoagulant administration

159. How is the knee most commonly supported post-operatively? By a

    A Thomas splint
    B plaster cylinder
    C plaster backslab
    D Robert Jones bandage

160. What are the special post-operative exercises taught by the physiotherapist known as:

    A passive
    B quadriceps
    C orthopaedic
    D active

Answers overleaf

157. **D**   62%

The meniscus is the half moon shaped cartilage in the knee joint between the head of the tibia and the condyles of the femur. Excision is called meniscectomy.

158. **C**   44%

All pre-operative preparation is important to prevent post-operative complications, but the tragic results of infection entering bone, such as permanent crippling, mean that extra precautions are taken to reduce the danger. Skin preparation is one of the measures which nurses are responsible for.

159. **D**   47%

The knee needs to be splinted and supported during the early healing stage, but easily accessible to the physiotherapist for carrying out exercises. The Robert Jones bandage, three alternate layers of orthopaedic wool and crepe bandage applied the full length of the leg gives this kind of support.

160. **B**   29%

Quadriceps exercises are taught and encouraged as these strengthen and support the knee joint. Active and passive exercises are general, not specific, exercises and applicable to any patient who is immobilised.

Mrs Walker has a ruptured fallopian tube due to an ectopic pregnancy. She is very shocked.

161. Which of the following is the average circulatory blood volume:

    A   3 litres
    B   5 litres
    C   7 litres
    D   9 litres

162. Which of the following will Mrs Walker exhibit:

    A   high temperature, bounding pulse
    B   high blood pressure, low temperature
    C   stertorous respirations, low blood pressure
    D   thready pulse, low blood pressure

163. Which type of shock will Mrs Walker present with:

    A   normovolaemic
    B   hypovolaemic
    C   anaphylactic
    D   neurogenic

164. In which position should Mrs Walker be nursed:

    A   recumbent with one pillow
    B   with head of the bed elevated
    C   semi-prone to protect her airway
    D   semi-prone with the foot of the bed elevated

Answers overleaf

161. B 74%

The normal blood volume in an adult is 5 litres. This does vary with size and weight and can be estimated approximately per kilogram of weight.

162. D 78%

Haemorrhage, excessive loss of blood from the circulation, results in the condition of hypovolaemic shock. There is insufficient blood in the circulation to carry the necessary oxygen and nutrients around the body. The decrease in circulating blood volume results in a low blood pressure (hypotension) and along with this the patient develops a rapid weak pulse (tachycardia) as the heart tries to compensate for the decreased blood volume by beating more rapidly. The patient also increases the respiratory rate in an attempt to increase the oxygen content of the blood, this is known as air hunger.

163. B 57%

Mrs Walker will have suffered loss of blood due to the rupturing of the fallopian tube. She will therefore be hypovolaemic. A means the normal amount of blood - this does not cause shock. C and D refer to other conditions causing shock. Anaphylactic shock is an allergic reaction which results in sudden vasodilation and a sudden need for blood to circulate in the peripheral blood vessels. Neurogenic shock arises when the nervous system is overstimulated, e.g. by a sudden fright.

164. A 81%

It is important in the condition of shock to maintain blood circulation between the heart and brain so the patient is nursed lying flat in a recumbent position. If a patient is vomiting or unable to maintain his airway he may be placed in a semi-prone position, but not in the case of Mrs Walker who is conscious.

Mrs Smith, a widow, is admitted for a pelvic floor repair. She has a severe prolapse which will require amputation of the cervix.

165. Which of the following is a possible indirect cause of uterine prolapse:

   A   stress incontinence
   B   chronic bronchitis
   C   excessive dietary roughage
   D   long working hours

166. Which of the following is a useful post-operative assessment of bladder tone:

   A   the amount of drainage is above 200 mls every 3 hours
   B   fluid intake is satisfactory and recorded accurately
   C   urine is passed naturally without pain or discomfort
   D   the amount in the bladder after micturition is less than 50 mls

167. Mrs Smith is advised to avoid heavy lifting post-operatively because

   A   the prolapse cannot recur but she should ensure that her muscle tone recovers
   B   the prolapse could recur, but avoiding lifting will reduce the likelihood
   C   bed rest will have resulted in muscular weakness
   D   she may develop haemorrhoids due to pelvic muscle strain

168. Protrusion of the cervix through the vagina is termed

   A   procidentia
   B   colpoperineorrhaphy
   C   colporrhaphy
   D   proctocele

Answers overleaf

165. B   23%

Coughing raises intra-abdominal pressure and persistent coughing can result in a weakened pelvic floor. The operation is usually carried out during a remission of bronchitis.
A is an effect not a cause.
C is not a cause of prolapse, in fact it would help reduce the incidence of constipation which can be a cause of prolapse.
D has no influence.

166. D   15%

This "residual urine" is indicative of resumption of adequate urethral micturition and bladder emptying.
A merely indicates functioning kidneys.
B is no indicator of bladder and voiding functions.
C - urinary output is dependent on fluid intake. This statement gives no indication that the bladder is emptied at micturition.

167. B   62%

With sensible muscle strengthening exercises and lack of strain the likelihood of a prolapse recurring can be reduced. The cervix is often ulcerated if procidentia has been long established.
Prolapse of the uterus can recur even though the cervix is amputated.
Haemorrhoids are not due to pelvic floor damage.

168. A   48%

When the cervix protrudes through the vagina as a result of uterine prolapse, this is termed procidentia.
A colporrhapy involves suturing of the vagina, a colpoperineorrhaphy also includes suturing of the perineum and a proctocele (or rectocele) arises when part of the rectum herniates into the vagina.

Mrs Taylor went to see her own doctor after palpating a lump in her right breast. She was admitted to hospital and taken to theatre for a simple mastectomy following a diagnosis of breast carcinoma.

169. Which of the following are some of the hormones responsible for mammary gland growth at puberty:

   A   oestrogen, oxytocin
   B   prolactin, oxytocin
   C   oestrogen, progesterone
   D   oxytocin, progesterone

170. Why is a wound drain inserted at the time of operation? To minimise

   A   oedema
   B   infection
   C   haemorrhage
   D   haematoma

171. How does breast cancer metastasise? By

   A   cells being transmitted to other parts of the body by blood and lymph
   B   parts of the tumour breaking off and moving to other parts
   C   the tumour secreting an exudate
   D   an infection in the lymphatic system

172. Which of the following psychological factors is *most* important when discharged:

   A   plenty of reading material to keep her mind occupied
   B   being able to wear her own clothes over the prosthesis
   C   plenty of visitors to talk to at home
   D   getting about and talking to other people

Answers overleaf

169. C   36%

Oxytocin causes the uterus to contract whilst prolactin is related to breast milk formation. It is oestrogen and progesterone which influence breast development during puberty.

170. D   36%

Drainage of the wound helps the prevention of haematoma and swelling.
This is important because the skin flaps must be allowed to adhere firmly to the chest wall to aid healing and prevent wound breakdown.

171. A   75%

The spread of breast cancer to other parts of the body (usually spinal metastases) arises because the blood and lymphatic fluid carries cells from the breast to distant organs.

172. B   67%

After mastectomy women are acutely aware of the fact that their body image has altered so the ability to wear their own clothes over the prosthesis is psychologically very important. A, C and D are relevant, but B must take priority.

Mrs Willow, a 24 year old housewife with a six week history of amenorrhoea, had severe abdominal pain about two hours prior to admission. Her diagnosis was ruptured right tubal pregnancy and a right salpingectomy was carried out. She gave up work as a staff nurse on a gynaecology ward six months ago.

173. Which of the following *best* describes Mrs Willow:

    A very shocked due to loss of blood
    B resting quietly to avoid an inevitable abortion
    C needing immediate dilatation and curettage to remove retained products of conception
    D needing drugs to cause uterine contractions

174. What will the nursing care plan be primarily based upon? A knowledge of

    A gynaecological nursing
    B abdominal operations
    C accidental abortions
    D Mrs Willow's needs and problems

175. What is meant by the term "evaluation of Mrs Willow's nursing care plan". To

    A determine the effectiveness of care given
    B record nursing care as planned in the Kardex
    C determine the priorities of care
    D assess the patient's initial problems

176. Which of the following is the *best* approach as Mrs Willow has worked as a trained nurse:

    A she may not require explanations of her care
    B her husband will be allowed special visiting privileges
    C she should be told when to expect a normal period
    D nurses must take extra care over what they say and do

173. A 43%

When a fallopian tube ruptures the blood vessels in its walls are also torn and there is bleeding into the peritoneum. Ruptured ectopic pregnancy is a surgical emergency as the patient may die from irreversible shock.
B - her pregnancy has already aborted into the peritoneal cavity.
C - dilatation and curettage are appropriate in incomplete abortion of a uterine pregnancy.
D - as the foetus is not in the uterus there would be little point in causing uterine contractions.

174. D 69%

Principles of care will need to be considered in these circumstances but Mrs Willow's individual needs require prime consideration. Her care plan should aim to meet her specific needs whilst incorporating gynaecological nursing principles.

175. A 44%

To "evaluate" means to consider what is of value, therefore by determining which nursing actions were effective or ineffective, one is evaluating Mrs Willow's care plan.

176. C 17%

A - patients should always be entitled to an explanation so that they know what is happening to them. Patients who are shocked are often unable to think rationally; knowledge should never be presumed.
B - visiting should not be considered a privilege but an important part of meeting patients' needs in hospital. Many people are unable to visit at "set" hospital times and ward staff should always be prepared to meet requests for alternative arrangements.
C - shedding of the lining of the uterus occurs following the termination of pregnancy.
D - nurses should always take care over what they say and do.

Mrs Brown is a 44 year old lady with two children in their early teens. She is admitted to hospital for investigations of her menorrhagia.

177. **Menorrhagia is**

    A inter-menstrual bleeding
    B excessive bleeding at menstruation
    C post-menopausal bleeding
    D painful menstruation

178. **The most common cause of menorrhagia is**

    A narrow cervix
    B endometriosis
    C intra-uterine contraception
    D middle age

179. **If Mrs Brown had a sudden severe loss of blood her**

    A blood pressure would fall and pulse rate increase
    B blood pressure would increase and pulse rate increase
    C blood pressure would increase and pulse rate decrease
    D blood pressure and pulse rate would show no noticeable change

180. **On Mrs Brown's return home her children should be**

    A asked to avoid disturbing their mother by being quiet in the house
    B encouraged to participate in household tasks
    C discouraged from enquiring about the nature of their mothers illness
    D sent on holiday to relatives to give mother a break

Answers overleaf

177. B   58%

Inter-menstrual and post-menopausal bleeding (bleeding between the menstrual period and after the menopause) warrants further medical investigation as both are abnormal. Painful menstruation is termed dysmenorrhoea.

178. B   34%

Thickening of the lining of the uterus or endometriosis is the commonest cause of menorrhagia.

179. A   66%

Whenever the body loses a considerable volume of blood the pressure exerted on the blood vessel walls will decrease. In an attempt to maintain adequate blood supply to the tissues the heart rate will increase, hence hypotension and tachycardia occur as a result of haemorrhage.

180. B   59%

Mrs Brown's children are in their early teens and therefore could be expected to help around the house whilst their mother recuperates. A, C and D are not realistic courses of action.

STATE ENROLMENT WRITTEN ASSESMENT TECHNIQUE

1. POINTS TO REMEMBER

Objective test examinations are intended to cover a large part of the syllabus, and it is unlikely that you will be able to answer all of the 60 questions easily. It is therefore wise to be prepared for the fact that there may be a small number of questions that you are unable to answer and you should not allow this to spoil your concentration during the examination.

Read the instructions *carefully* before you begin.

The time allocation of 1½ hours for a 60 item examination may seem generous, but it is intended as 'thinking' time, enabling you to choose the correct answer after careful, reasoned thought. There is only *one* correct answer to each question, but if there seems to you to be more than one possible answer, then read the stem of the question again. There will be some information there to guide you. For example, "Which one of the following is the *most* important" indicates that all four alternatives could be important but one has priority over the rest. Similarly, "Which one of the following must be reported immediately" suggests that all four alternatives may be significant and ought to be reported, but that one deserves *immediate* action.

Note that it is possible to alter your choice of answer but you *cannot* then revert to your original choice, so think carefully before making your decision.

2. MARKING THE COMPUTER SHEET

Only a Grade B (soft) pencil must be used.

Enter your candidate number like this:-

CANDIDATE NUMBER **0 2 7 1**

Write your
CANDIDATE NUMBER
in the boxes provided
AND mark the same
figure in the column
below each box
Mark the number
thus: —

When answering a question, mark the letter corresponding to the answer you consider correct. There is only one correct answer.

e.g. If you consider the answer to question 1 to be   a)
      mark thus: using heavy
      pencil lines.

To cancel an answer fill in
the bottom of the square thus:
and re-mark the correct letter.

Do not use a rubber.
It is not possible in the
case of question 4 to
return to a) and re-mark it.

	a	b	c	d
1	▬			
2				
3				
4	▬			▬
5				
6				
7				
8				
9				
10				
11				
12				
13				

You should attempt all 60 questions as marks are not deducted for incorrect answers.

PRACTICE EXAM INSTRUCTIONS

This practice examination for the written assessment has been compiled, as far as possible, to correspond with the range of topics and degree of difficulty which one could expect to find in the SEN Final Examination. Having completed the preceding 180 questions, you will be familiar with the range of topics, but the degree of difficulty of the practice examination questions falls within the range 20% - 72%. The very difficult and very easy questions have been omitted in order to provide a realistic examination.

There are 60 questions and the time allowed is 1½ hours. Do not spend more than the allotted time.

Try to work under conditions which resemble those of the final examination.
Do not refer to books, notes or speak to other persons.
Do not smoke - no smoking is allowed during the final examination.

Choose a time when you will be free from distractions and undisturbed, in a well-lit location. A watch or clock should be easily visible.

Answers, with explanations and degree of difficulty (as a %) are to be found on page 109. The pass mark is 50%, i.e. 30 or more correct.

Questions 1 - 4 refer to the following case study.

Mr Burns has just returned from theatre after having an emergency tracheostomy due to an obstruction in his upper respiratory tract. He is 54 and lives alone.

1. Whilst Mr Burns is recovering from surgery, in which position will he be nursed:

    A   upright
    B   supine
    C   semi-prone
    D   prone

2. Whilst carrying out tracheal aspiration, you should apply suction

    A   only when inserting the catheter during expiration
    B   intermittently while inserting the catheter
    C   intermittently while removing the catheter
    D   only when removing the catheter on inspiration

3. When may Mr Burns begin to eat and drink:

    A   when bowel sounds are heard
    B   two days post-operatively
    C   when he has passed flatus
    D   when his swallowing reflex returns

4. In the immediate post-operative period the *most* important nursing care is

    A   chest physiotherapy, observations of skin and pulse
    B   observations of pulse, respirations and temperature
    C   chest physiotherapy, observations of pulse and respirations
    D   observations of skin, respirations and pulse

Questions 5 - 8 refer to the following case study.

Mrs Margaret Chorley, aged 23 years, is 3 months pregnant. She has been married 2 years and this is her first pregnancy. She is admitted with lower abdominal pain and slight vaginal blood loss.

5. Which of the following would be the aim of Mrs Chorley's nursing care:

    A maintenance of bedrest initially
    B prevention of an inevitable abortion
    C reassurance of a successful pregnancy in the future
    D early mobilisation to prevent the complications of bedrest

6. Which of the following statements describes an inevitable abortion:

    A slight vaginal blood loss and closed cervix
    B abdominal pain and heavy vaginal blood loss
    C passage of products of conception per vagina
    D severe abdominal pain and heavy brown discharge per vagina

7. Several hours after Mrs Chorley's admission her pulse rate increases from 90 to 120 beats/minute. The *most* likely reason would be

    A anxiety
    B pain
    C haemorrhage
    D shock

8. Mrs Chorley has a further bleed per vagina and it is decided to take her to theatre for evacuation of uterus. The reason for this is

    A prevention of haemorrhage and infection
    B legal termination of pregnancy
    C examination to determine competency of cervix
    D prevention of uterine prolapse and haemorrhage

Questions 9 - 12 refer to the following case study.

Mrs Harriet Stoves, a 72 year old retired post mistress, is seen at the Outpatients Department where a diagnosis of myxoedema (hypothyroidism) is made. She lives alone in a two-bedroomed cottage.

9. Which of the following signs and symptoms are likely:

   A   constipation, slow pulse, severe anxiety and indigestion
   B   hoarse voice, coarse skin, slow pulse and weight gain
   C   hypotension, sweating, coarse skin and diarrhoea
   D   tachycardia, mental dullness, poor memory and constipation

10. **Thyroxine is**

   A   started with high doses and given for life
   B   given in small doses for several months prior to surgery
   C   initially given in small doses and given for life
   D   given in increasingly large doses until recovery occurs

11. **Why would Mrs Stoves' temperature be recorded regularly? Because**

   A   her low metabolic rate would mask the signs and symptoms of infection
   B   the drug regime renders her much more susceptible to infection
   C   the risk of chest infection and deep vein thrombosis are increased
   D   her low metabolic rate could lead to hypothermia

12. **Which is the main reason for Mrs Stoves being referred to the Health Visitor:**

   A   her therapy requires supervision and her home conditions need monitoring
   B   she will eventually require admission to a long term ward for the elderly
   C   all patients over the age of 70 years are referred in this manner
   D   her diet and hygiene need monitoring and supervision

Questions 13 - 16 refer to the following case study.

Mrs Mary Brown is having a second unit of whole blood transfused when a patchy erythema is observed on her skin. Her pulse is 90 beats/minute, blood pressure 110/65 mmHg, respiration 22 per minute.

13. Which of the following statements is the *best* explanation of this situation:

   A the respiratory rate suggests circulatory overloading
   B a mild skin reaction is to be expected and is insignificant
   C a life threatening situation is present which indicates mismatched transfusion
   D probably an allergic reaction, but more serious complications are possible

14. The nurse caring for Mrs Brown should initially

   A stop the transfusion
   B seek urgent help
   C stay with the patient
   D record her temperature

15. Which of the following nursing observations are *most* suitable during a blood transfusion:

   A hourly pulse and blood pressure, 4 hourly temperature throughout the whole transfusion period
   B hourly pulse, blood pressure, temperature and respiratory rate throughout the whole transfusion period
   C ¼ hourly pulse and blood pressure for first ½ hour of each new unit and then hourly temperature and blood pressure
   D ½ hourly pulse throughout transfusion and 2 hourly temperature, blood pressure and respiratory rate

16. The infusion site should be regularly checked because

   A a blood clot may block the giving set, stopping the flow
   B the intravenous needle may penetrate the vein wall
   C local irritation of the site is common during transfusion of blood
   D spasm of the vein may seriously reduce transfusion effectiveness

Questions 17 - 21 refer to the following case study.

Mr Arthur Cunningham, aged 41 years is admitted to hospital complaining of severe headache and weakness of his right side. Sub-arachnoid haemorrhage is suspected.

17. Which of the following will confirm the diagnosis:

  A lumbar puncture
  B skull X-ray
  C full neurological examination
  D carotid angiogram

18. Which of the following is the most likely cause of sub-arachnoid haemorrhage:

  A cerebral thrombosis
  B fractured skull
  C cerebral haemorrhage
  D ruptured aneurysm

19. Where does the bleeding occur during a sub-arachnoid haemorrhage:

  A above the arachnoid, above the pia
  B beneath the dura, above the arachnoid
  C above the dura, beneath the arachnoid
  D beneath the arachnoid, above the pia

20. Which of the following actual problems will be identified when assessing Mr Cunningham's needs and planning his care:

  A enforced immobility
  B inability to maintain airway
  C dehydration and sweating
  D urinary incontinence

Questions 21 - 24 refer to the following case study.

Mrs Widdows has been admitted for a cholecystectomy and exploration of the common bile duct.

21. Cholelithiasis is

    A a substance released continuously before meals
    B the presence of gall stones
    C a hormone secreted by gall bladder cells
    D a substance responsible for gall bladder emptying

22. Which of the following best describes Mrs Widdows' post-operative nursing care plan:

    A compare the information collected with the normal activities
    B select nursing actions to meet objectives of care
    C modify the care plan as Mrs Widdows' problems change
    D give the proposed nursing care as prescribed

23. Prior to removal of a T-tube, it is most important that

    A sedation is given
    B the jaundice has subsided
    C the common bile duct is radiologically patent
    D bile has ceased draining from the tube

24. The T-tube generally remains in place for

    A 2 - 3 days
    B 4 - 5 days
    C 7 - 10 days
    D 12 - 14 days

Questions 25 - 28 refer to the following case study.

Mrs Taylor aged 45 is admitted to your ward with a provisional diagnosis of pernicious anaemia.

25.   Which of the following is lacking in pernicious anaemia:

   A   extrinsic factor
   B   intrinsic factor
   C   ascorbic acid
   D   ferrous sulphate

26.   Which of the following is a complication of pernicious anaemia:

   A   myocardial infarction
   B   spinal cord degeneration
   C   beri-beri
   D   malabsorption syndrome

27.   Which of the following investigations will confirm the diagnosis:

   A   a Schilling test
   B   a pentagastrin test
   C   haemoglobin estimation
   D   erythrocyte sedimentation rate (E.S.R.)

28.   Which of the following would be the drug of choice in the treatment of Mrs Taylor:

   A   Imferon
   B   cyanocobalamine
   C   Sorbitol
   D   Mercaptamine

29. Which of the following will result after an abdo-perineal excision of rectum:

    A temporary ileostomy
    B permanent colostomy
    C permanent ileostomy
    D temporary colostomy

30. Why is skin care needed around an ileostomy? Because

    A ileostomy appliances need changing twice daily
    B vitamin malabsorption impairs skin regeneration
    C digestive enzymes cause excoriation
    D the appliance adhesive irritates the stoma

31. When explaining to a junior nurse the meaning of cachexia, which of the following definitions applies:

    A bad breath
    B loss of appetite
    C malnutrition and wasting
    D alopecia

32. Which of the following statements about intestinal obstruction is true:

    A the small bowel only is affected
    B the obstruction is mechanical or paralytic in nature
    C surgical treatment is always required
    D obstructions are always acute in nature

33. A woman with untreated gonorrhoea is in danger of giving birth to a baby with

   A infected eyes
   B congenital syphilis
   C vaginal thrush
   D gonococcal salpingitis

34. Which of the following activities should be organised if a patient is pyrexial on the first day following a total abdominal hysterectomy:

   A alert the physiotherapist to the patient's condition
   B take a wound swab for culture of organism
   C ensure a speedier intravenous infusion rate
   D withhold oral fluids until seen by a doctor

35. Which of the following is the usual management for a patient with Hodgkin's disease:

   A high protein diet
   B antibiotic regime
   C chemotherapy
   D radical surgery

36. An infant weighing 3 Kg is prescribed 0.425 milligrams of a drug per Kg of body weight. The total amount of drug administered will be

   A 0.1275 mg
   B 1.275 mg
   C 12.75 mg
   D 127.5 mg

37. Initially, after a haematemesis of 600 mls., an adult patient will be treated by

   A emergency laparotomy
   B rest and nil orally
   C partial gastrectomy
   D gastro-enterostomy

38. Which of the following will prevent a febrile convulsion from occuring:

   A withholding fluids
   B lowering the body temperature
   C giving an anti-epileptic drug
   D barrier nursing

39. Following a Pott's fracture the patient will have difficulty

   A writing
   B chewing
   C bending
   D walking

40. Which of the following complications is particularly likely to occur following liver biopsy:

   A coma
   B vomiting
   C haemorrhage
   D haematuria

41. Which of the following is a long term complication of vagotomy and pyloroplasty:

    A   recurrence of ulceration
    B   explosive diarrhoea
    C   effortless vomiting
    D   dumping syndrome

42. Which of the following drugs would be prescribed for a patient who has mild jaundice and is scheduled for surgery in 10 days time:

    A   antibiotics
    B   iron
    C   vitamin K
    D   vitamin E

43. Which of the following conditions results in the blood pressure rising and the pulse rate falling:

    A   subdural haematoma
    B   hypovolaemia
    C   oligaemic shock
    D   liver failure

44. Which of the following is a correct definition of cardiac tamponade:

    A   fluid pressure in the pericardial sac restricting the heart
    B   a special pack always used in cardiac surgery
    C   pressure pads applied to the cardiac septum to prevent bleeding
    D   an electrode passed into the heart via a venous catheter

45. Which of the following observations is *most* significant when a patient has atrial fibrillation:

    A   blood pressure and pulse
    B   pulse and apex beat
    C   apex beat and blood pressure
    D   respirations and temperature

46. Why is a nasogastric tube in position post-operatively following vagotomy and pyloroplasty? To

    A   keep the stomach as empty as possible
    B   give nasogastric feeds 4 hourly
    C   inhibit secretion of gastric juices
    D   allow the stomach to rest

47. Prior to removing a chest drain you should instruct the patient to

    A   breathe slowly and shallowly
    B   expire and hold his breath
    C   breathe deeply and slowly
    D   inspire and hold his breath

48. Which of the following dietary regimes is suitable when a patient has chronic renal failure:

    A   low protein, low salt, low carbohydrate
    B   high protein, low fat, high carbohydrate
    C   low protein, low salt, high carbohydrate
    D   high protein, high fat, low carbohydrate

49. Why do patients with congestive cardiac failure develop oedema? Because

   A they have a raised serum potassium
   B they have a low level of plasma proteins
   C the output of antidiuretic hormone is increased
   D the venous pressure is raised

50. A middle aged woman had rheumatic fever as a child of 12. Which of the following diseases is she most likely to present with now:

   A infective carditis
   B Cushing's syndrome
   C mitral stenosis
   D osteomyelitis

51. A patient with a hiatus hernia will be advised to

   A lie down for at least half an hour after meals
   B sleep well supported by pillows at night
   C take antacids before meals and first thing in the morning
   D begin a low fat diet immediately

52. Which of the following potential problems are you likely to highlight when a patient suffers from acute ulcerative colitis:

   A pressure sores, constipation and reluctance to eat
   B pyschological disturbance and urinary tract infection
   C reluctance to eat, dehydration and pressure sores
   D sore mouth, incontinence and diarrhoea

53. **Why may a cerebrovascular accident occur in patients with damaged heart valves? Because**

A there is an increase in serum cholesterol and thrombosis may occur
B vegetations can travel in the blood stream and cause embolism
C the blood pressure rises rapidly and is difficult to control
D platelets adhere to the damaged valves causing bleeding

54. **A steroid retention enema will**

A produce a local anti-inflammatory effect
B produce a local anti-coagulant effect
C increase muscle tone in the bowel wall
D cause evacuation of the rectum

55. **Why will intravenous therapy be erected in the Accident and Emergency Department when a patient has a severe myocardial infarction? To**

A correct shock and introduce a venous pressure line
B provide a route for the injection of intravenous drugs
C prevent dehydration and potassium imbalance
D promote circulatory function and maintain blood pressure

56. **Which of the following may be used in the treatment of epistaxis:**

A Egometrine
B Erepsin
C Ephedrine
D Eraldin

57. Which of the following drugs may cause agranulocytosis:

   A codeine
   B clonidine hydrochloride
   C Cyclimorph
   D chloramphenicol

58. Which of the following blood groups is safest when given in an emergency without grouping and cross-matching:

   A AB+
   B AB-
   C O+
   D O-

59. Which of the following drugs induces diuresis:

   A spironolactone
   B slow K
   C suxamethonium chloride
   D sulphadimidine

60. The most likely sign that will be present from cytotoxic therapy will be

   A apoplexy
   B alopecia
   C aphasia
   D aphagia

END OF PRACTICE EXAMINATION

PRACTICE EXAM ANSWERS

1. **A   46%**

    Mr Burns would be nursed in an upright position to facilitate adequate breathing. His airway is maintained by the tracheostomy tube so he does not need to be in a semi-prone position. Neither will he be placed in a supine position (flat on his back) or in a prone position (flat on his front).

2   **C   48%**

    Tracheal suction is carried out to remove excess secretions from the lungs. It is important to insert the catheter without suction so that it does not adhere to any part of the tracheal lining and then to apply suction as the catheter is withdrawn. Chest physiotherapy immediately prior to suction is especially beneficial.

3. **D   54%**

    Mr Burns will be able to commence eating and drinking when his swallowing reflex has returned. He can take fluids as tolerated, usually within several hours of the operation. There has been no direct handling of the bowel so bowel sounds should be present anyway.

4. **C   41%**

    Chest physiotherapy is extremely important to Mr Burns in order to prevent the complication of chest infection. Observations of pulse are important in case of haemorrhage. Observations of respirations are important to ensure adequate oxygen exchange and to be aware of any possible obstruction to the respiratory tract or displacement of the tube.

5. **A   49%**

    As the patient is suffering a possible threatened abortion, bedrest must be maintained in order to safeguard the pregnancy if at all possible.
    B is not possible; C is the responsibility of the doctor and D is a dangerous practice in this particular situation.

6.　C　22%

An abortion is inevitable when there is evidence that the pregnancy is to be lost and C gives the best explanation of this.

7.　C　56%

On admission this patient was suffering pain, she was anxious and her pulse rate was 90 beats/minute. The reason for the increase in pulse rate is most likely to be haemorrhage as that is a typical outcome of this situation. The heart rate increases in an effort to keep the body supplied with sufficient oxygen despite the lowered blood volume.

8.　A　38%

The reason for the evacuation of the uterus is that following an inevitable abortion the products of conception may be retained in the uterus, therefore infection may occur and uterine contraction will be inhibited leading to haemorrhage.

9.　B　42%

Hypothyroidism is a condition in which the secretion of thyroxine (thyroid hormone) is reduced. As thyroxine is required by all cells for metabolism, the patient's signs and symptoms all indicate a low metabolic rate.
Severe anxiety, diarrhoea, sweating and tachycardia are not common features of this condition. They are, however, common in thyrotoxicosis.

10.   **C   51%**

Mrs Stoves has probably had a low output of thyroxine for quite a long period of time in order for her body to undergo the changes seen in myxoedema. If her replacement hormone (thyroxine) were given in high doses the sudden impact on her physiology might be more than her body could cope with and have dangerous consequences. 'Small doses' is reasonable but this lady will not require surgery. Surgery is a more common treatment for an overactive gland where some of it can be removed.
C is the correct answer as she needs to adjust gradually to the drug. As it is a replacement hormone (due to her natural lack of it), it will therefore need to be given for life.

11.   **D   61%**

Hypothermia is a risk in the elderly and it is very typically associated with hypothyroidism as the sufferer cannot generate her own heat.

12.   **A   71%**

Mrs Stoves must take her medication correctly and with increasing doses this can be rather complicated. As she lives alone it is important to ensure that she can manage and that she is going to be warm enough during the winter.
There is no indication that hospital admission on a long-term basis is likely as myxoedema can be controlled.

13.   **D   62%**

In view of the relatively stable signs the rash would indicate an allergic reaction which is probable. The nurse however must not rule out the possibility of serious complications such as a mismatched transfusion and will be alert for any further change in Mrs Brown's condition.

14. **A** 71%

In view of the fact that this may be a serious complication such as mismatched transfusion, in order to be safe the nurse should stop the transfusion whilst medical staff are notified and recordings of temperature taken.

15. **C** 27%

The danger period is the start of each new unit when any serious complication is likely to show up therefore C is correct. Ideally nursing staff should observe the patient very carefully for the first few minutes of each unit of blood.

16. **B** 69%

B is the reason that any infusion site should be checked regularly. A and D would not be identified by examination of the infusion site and C is incorrect.

17. **A** 61%

During a sub-arachnoid haemorrhage bleeding occurs into the cerebrospinal fluid. Because of this, the normally clear fluid will appear blood-stained when a lumbar puncture is performed and will confirm the suspected diagnosis. B and C would not confirm the diagnosis, and D could be dangerous.

18. **D** 43%

The most likely cause of a sub-arachnoid haemorrhage is a ruptured aneurysm. A weakness in the blood vessel wall causes it to distend and eventually to burst. A and C are causes of cerebrovascular accidents whilst B is more likely to result in a blood clot beneath the dura mater (a sub-dural haematoma).

19. **D** 36%

As the name implies, a *sub*-arachnoid haemorrhage results in bleeding beneath the arachnoid mater into the cerebrospinal fluid in the sub-arachnoid space.
The order of meninges (from the brain towards the skull) is pia mater arachnoid mater dura mater therefore D is the correct response.

20. **A   44%**

Mr Cunningham will be nursed on complete bed rest on admission therefore "enforced immobility" is an actual (i.e. existing) problem to be considered when planning his nursing care.

B is incorrect as consciousness has not been lost. There is no indication that C and D are actual problems; they are potential problems (i.e. could arise in the future) to be considered and avoided if possible.

21. **B   47%**

Cholelithiasis is a term used to describe the presence of stones in the biliary tract.

22. **C   21%**

No care plan can be drawn up in advance or without the patient being involved. Therefore, post-operatively, Mrs Widdows' care plan should be modified according to how she is responding in the post-operative period.

Each time a new problem arises the care plan must include the problem, the aim of care and how that care will be given.

23. **C   70%**

A T-tube is usually inserted in the common bile duct if there has been exploration of the duct or a stone removed. The T-tube serves as a safety valve through which excess bile can drain while the intestine is adjusting to receiving a continuous flow of bile. It also prevents the back flow of bile to the liver and leakage into the peritoneal cavity. Amounts of bile drainage over 1000 mls/24 hours should alert the nurse to the possibility of ductal obstruction below the location of the tube and the doctor would need to be informed promptly. A decrease in the bile output accompanied by a return of colour to the stool is indicative of a normal bile flow. It is important that there is a free flow of bile into the intestines before the tube is removed and this is checked by a T-tube cholangiogram.

24. **B   68%**

After 4 - 5 days the T-tube is clamped for 1 - 2 hours before and after meals. If there is no pain and nausea and no increase in bile loss into the bag, this indicates that the bile is emptying into the duodenum. The T-tube should remain in position for 24 hours after the cholangiogram to allow the dye to drain.

25. **B   60%**

The extrinsic factor is in the food we eat known as vitamin B_{12}.
The intrinsic factor present in gastric juice is necessary for the absorption of vitamin B_1 in the terminal ileum. Ascorbic acid is vitamin C and deficiency causes scurvy.
Ferrous sulphate is iron and is used in the treatment of iron deficiency anaemia.

26. **B   23%**

Pernicious anaemia may cause neurological damage. The patient may complain of tingling in the extremities and clumsiness of fine movement - this is peripheral neuropathy and spinal cord damage may follow.
C is lack of vitamin B_1 which causes pain from neuritis, paralysis, muscular weakness, progressive oedema, mental deterioration and heart failure.
A is due to disease within the coronary arteries.
D is unrelated to pernicious anaemia and is caused by lesions of the small intestines, lack of digestive enzymes or bile salts, and surgical operations.

27.   **A   47%**

The Schilling test definitely confirms pernicious anaemia as it measures the amount of B_{12} excreted in the urine. Pernicious anaemia is due to lack of vitamin B_{12}, the cells are large and may still contain a nucleus.
Studies of haemoglobin will confirm that the patient has anaemia but not the cause. Normal haemoglobin is 13.4 - 17.0 g/dl in men and 11.4 - 15.0 g/dl in women. The erythrocyte sedimentation rate (E.S.R.) is usually raised in infection.
A pentagastrin test is used to estimate the amount of hydrochloric acid in the stomach. Deficiency of hydrochloric acid (achlorhydria) may be a cause of pernicious anaemia but does not confirm diagnosis.

28. **B 66%**

Cyanocobalamine is vitamin B_{12} which is lacking in pernicious anaemia.
Imferon or iron dextran is used to treat iron deficiency anaemia as is Sorbitol, a drug which contains 5% iron.
Mercaptamine (Cytamin) is an antidote used in cases of paracetamol poisoning.
When vitamin B_{12} is given to the patient the intramuscular route is used. As the patient has no intrinsic factor in the stomach the drug would not be absorbed if given orally.

29. **B 44%**

If the rectum has been excised then a permanent stoma must be fashioned so that faeces can be excreted. The colon will be brought out onto the abdominal wall, thus B, permanent colostomy is correct.

30. **C 54%**

Ileostomy appliances only require changing if there is a leakage. The appliances should fit the stoma well but not cause irritation.
Vitamin absorption should occur in the jejunum and therefore is unaffected although the patient may be given additional vitamin C to aid in wound healing.
It is the digestive enzymes present in the liquid faeces which will excoriate the skin around the stoma if leakage should occur.

31. **C 34%**

Halitosis means bad breath; anorexia is loss of appetite and alopecia means hair loss.
Cachexia refers to the extreme wasting and emaciation which occurs when patients have terminal cancer.

32. **B 23%**

It is possible for obstruction to occur in the large bowel; surgical treatment is not always required and the obstruction could be chronic in nature. B then is correct - either paralysis of the intestine or a mechanical problem (i.e. physical obstruction) will cause the obstruction in intestinal movement.

33. **A** 30%

During childbirth the baby will come into contact with the gonococcal infection and as a result can suffer from an eye infection known as ophthalmia neonatorum.

34. **A** 29%

As the pyrexia has arisen on the first post-operative day a chest infection is the most likely cause and initially the physiotherapist should be alerted.
It is rather early for a wound infection to be the cause of the pyrexia whilst options C and D are not relevant under the circumstances described.

35. **C** 51%

Hodgkin's disease is a malignant disease which causes enlargement of the lymph nodes and affects the bone marrow. As it is a generalised disease of the lymph system it is treated by chemotherapy not radical surgery.
Antibiotics are not required unless there is an infection. Patients can usually manage a normal diet so do not require a high protein diet.

36. **B** 56%

$$0.425 \text{ mg per Kg body weight} = 0.425 \times 3$$
$$= 1.275 \text{ mg}$$

37. **B** 62%

After a haematemesis the patient will be weak and anaemic and therefore not in a fit state for surgery, so rest and nil orally is the initial treatment which may also be preparation for elective surgery. Immediate surgery is only performed when there has been a peptic perforation.

38. **B** 46%

To prevent a febrile convulsion cooling measures should be taken, such as liberal fluids to drink, sponging the skin frequently and removing excessive bedclothes from the patient. Care must be taken not to lower body temperature too rapidly as this would cause the patient to collapse.

39. D 30%

A Pott's fracture involves the fibula therefore walking would be difficult.

40. C 54%

The liver is a very vascular organ and therefore haemorrhage is a likely and serious complication following biopsy.

41. D 60%

The dumping syndrome may occur following vagotomy and pyloroplasty or gastro-enterostomy. Food is literally "dumped" into the jejunum which distends, and there is a rapid withdrawal of water from the circulating blood volume. This decreases the circulatory blood volume producing palpitations, fainting, perspiration and extreme weakness.

42. C 64%

Bile secreted by the liver is essential in the gut if fat soluble vitamin K is to be digested and absorbed. Once absorbed the vitamin K is transported to the liver which then produces clotting substances. As the patient has jaundice her liver function or ability to absorb vitamin K may be impaired which will result in an increased bleeding tendency. Therefore replacement vitamin K is given pre-operatively.

43. A 44%

A haematoma beneath the dura mater would result in pressure symptoms arising within the cranial cavity causing bradycardia and hypertension.
This is an emergency situation and medical help must be summoned.
Hypovolaemic and oligaemic shock would mean low blood volume and produce hypotension.
Liver failure which may be acute or chronic, results in a raised level of waste products e.g. ammonia.

44. A 26%

Cardiac tamponade is an acute (sudden) filling of the pericardial sac with blood or fluid which interferes with diastolic filling. It can occur from blunt or penetrating chest injuries, and sometimes following myocardial infarction. This is an emergency situation.

45.   B   69%

All the observations are important but the recording of the apex beat with the pulse for a full minute will show any deficiency between the beating of the heart and the pulse rate. In atrial fibrillation the atria may beat faster than the ventricles and beat irregularly.

46.   A   53%

It is important to keep the stomach empty; this allows and promotes healing and prevents vomiting post-operatively. 4 hourly tube feeds may not be part of post-operative management.

47.   D   51%

When removing a chest drain it is important to prevent air entering the pleural space. If John breathes in and holds his breath he is maintaining a high pressure in the lungs and therefore creating pressure between the two layers of pleura. This prevents air rushing into the pleural cavity as the tube is removed. The area must immediately be covered with an airtight dressing.

48.   C   42%

Because the kidneys cannot excrete waste products in chronic renal failure, the amount of protein and salt eaten must be restricted. (The end product of protein digestion is urea.) In order to provide sufficient calories for daily energy requirements a high carbohydrate diet is given.

49.   D   42%

Because of the generalised venous congestion which occurs in congestive heart failure the venous pressure is higher than normal. Fluid which would normally pass from the tissues into the bloodstream is not reabsorbed because of the high pressure in the veins and oedema results.

50.   C   57%

Damage to the mitral valve because of scarring resulting from past inflammation is likely to produce mitral stenosis (narrowing). Infective carditis is caused by many infections. Osteomyelitis is inflammation of bone and Cushing's syndrome is caused by excessive steroid levels in the bloodstream.

51.   **B   56%**

In hiatus hernia the weakened cardiac sphincter muscle at the entrance to the stomach allow stomach contents to flow backwards into the oesophagus.

A - the principle of treatment is to reduce regurgitation of food and stomach enzymes through the non-functioning cardiac sphincter. Lying down is strongly contra-indicated for at least two hours after meals.

B - this will reduce regurgitation. Sometimes patients are advised to put blocks under the head of the bed. C - antacids are often prescribed to be taken half an hour *after* meals and at bedtime. D - a low fat diet would not relieve the signs and symptoms of hiatus hernia.

52.   **C   72%**

Potential problems are those which the patient may not have on admission but could arise at some later time. Patients with diarrhoea will often associate this with food and therefore be reluctant to eat. Because of the diarrhoea the patient may well develop dehydration. Finally, patients with acute ulcerative colitis are generally very thin which will also make pressure sores a potential problem.

53.   **B   41%**

When the heart valves are damaged vegetations present on the valves can break loose and travel in the blood stream causing embolism. Cerebrovascular accidents can be caused by an emboli therefore patients should be observed for the possibility of this occurrence if it is known that they have mitral valve damage.

54.   **A   71%**

Retention enemata containing steroids are a common form of treatment when an anti-inflammatory effect on the bowel wall is required, for example when a patient has ulcerative colitis.

55.   **B   42%**

The patient requires a route for the injection of intravenous drugs because his condition may deteriorate, his veins collapse and serious complications develop. He may need intravenous sodium bicarbonate if he has a cardiac arrest or intravenous lignocaine in order to correct arrhythmias.

56.   C   67%

Egometrine is a drug used to cause contraction of the uterus after delivery to prevent or reduce haemorrhage.

Erepsin is an enzyme found in the alimentary tract aiding the digestion of protein.

Ephedrine is used as a nasal decongestant and causes constriction of blood vessels.

Eraldin is a drug used to correct cardiac dysrrhythmias.

57.   D   49%

Agranulocytosis means "absence of granulocytes" which are the white blood cells which help fight infection.

Codeine and cyclimorph are analgesics and clonidine hydrochlroide is an anti-hypertensive; these do not have the side effect of agranulocytosis.

Chloramphenicol is an antibiotic and can cause severe agranulocytosis which means that the patient is at risk from infection because of lowered body resistance. One early sign of this in at risk patients is a sore throat.

58.   D   32%

O Rhesus negative is the safest blood to give as there are no antigens present on the red cells to cause agglutination. Group O is known for this reason as the "Universal Donor".

59.   A   62%

Spironolactone is a diuretic.

Slow K is "Potassium Slow Release" Suxamethonium chloride is a muscle relaxant.

Sulphadimidine is a sulphonamide drug i.e. a bacteriostatic agent.

60.   B   68%

Apoplexy (a cerebrovascular disorder) is not a condition that results from cytotoxic therapy.

Alopecia is when the hair is lost and this is a possible physical change that the person may experience when receiving cytotoxic therapy.

Aphasia means loss of the ability to communicate by speaking, and is not related to cytotoxic therapy.

Aphagia is absence of swallowing which does not occur as a direct result of cytotoxic therapy.